MW01658412

FREE Study Skills DVD Offer

Dear Customer,

Thank you for your purchase from Mometrix! We consider it an honor and a privilege that you have purchased our product and we want to ensure your satisfaction.

As a way of showing our appreciation and to help us better serve you, we have developed a Study Skills DVD that we would like to give you for FREE. This DVD covers our *best practices* for getting ready for your exam, from how to use our study materials to how to best prepare for the day of the test.

All that we ask is that you email us with feedback that would describe your experience so far with our product. Good, bad, or indifferent, we want to know what you think!

To get your FREE Study Skills DVD, email freedvd@mometrix.com with *FREE STUDY SKILLS DVD* in the subject line and the following information in the body of the email:

- The name of the product you purchased.
- Your product rating on a scale of 1-5, with 5 being the highest rating.
- Your feedback. It can be long, short, or anything in between. We just want to know your impressions and experience so far with our product. (Good feedback might include how our study material met your needs and ways we might be able to make it even better. You could highlight features that you found helpful or features that you think we should add.)
- Your full name and shipping address where you would like us to send your free DVD.

If you have any questions or concerns, please don't hesitate to contact me directly.

Thanks again!

Sincerely,

Jay Willis
Vice President
jay.willis@mometrix.com
1-800-673-8175

Mometrix
TEST PREPARATION

HESI A^2 Practice Book 2020-2021

Two Full-Length HESI® Practice Exams for the HESI® Admission Assessment 5th Edition [Updated for the New Exam Review Outline]

Dear Future Exam Success Story

First of all, **THANK YOU** for purchasing Mometrix study materials!

Second, congratulations! You are one of the few determined test-takers who are committed to doing whatever it takes to excel on your exam. **You have come to the right place.** We developed these practice tests with one goal in mind: to deliver you the best possible approximation of the questions you will see on test day.

Standardized testing is one of the biggest obstacles on your road to success, which only increases the importance of doing well in the high-pressure, high-stakes environment of test day. Your results on this test could have a significant impact on your future, and these practice tests will give you the repetitions you need to build your familiarity and confidence with the test content and format to help you achieve your full potential on test day.

Your success is our success

We would love to hear from you! If you would like to share the story of your exam success or if you have any questions or comments in regard to our products, please contact us at **800-673-8175** or **support@mometrix.com**.

Thanks again for your business and we wish you continued success!

Sincerely,
The Mometrix Test Preparation Team

Written and edited by the Mometrix Exam Secrets Test Prep Team
Printed in the United States of America

TABLE OF CONTENTS

Practice Test #1

Reading Comprehension

Questions 1 to 8 pertain to the following passage:

Visual Perception

It is tempting to think that your eyes are simply mirrors that reflect whatever is in front of them. Researchers, however, have shown that your brain is constantly working to create the impression of a continuous, uninterrupted world.

For instance, in the last ten minutes, you have blinked your eyes around 200 times. You have probably not been aware of any of these interruptions in your visual world. Something you probably have not seen in a long time without the aid of a mirror is your nose. It is always right there, down in the bottom corner of your vision, but your brain filters it out so that you are not aware of your nose unless you purposefully look at it.

Nor are you aware of the artery that runs right down the middle of your retina. It creates a large blind spot in your visual field, but you never notice the hole it leaves. To see this blind spot, try the following: Cover your left eye with your hand. With your right eye, look at the O on the left. As you move your head closer to the O, the X will disappear as it enters the blind spot caused by your optical nerve.

O X

Your brain works hard to make the world look continuous!

1. The word <u>filters</u>, as used in this passage, most nearly means:

a. Alternates
b. Reverses
c. Ignores
d. Depends

2. The word <u>retina</u>, as used in this passage, most nearly means:

a. Optical illusion
b. Part of the eye
c. Pattern
d. Blindness

3. Which of the following statements can be inferred from this passage?

a. Not all animals' brains filter out information
b. Visual perception is not a passive process
c. Blind spots cause accidents
d. The eyes never reflect reality

4. What is the author's purpose for including the two letters near the end of the passage?

a. To demonstrate the blind spot in the visual field
b. To organize the passage
c. To transition between the last two paragraphs of the passage
d. To prove that the blind spot is not real

5. What is the main purpose of this passage?

a. To persuade the reader to pay close attention to blind spots
b. To explain the way visual perception works
c. To persuade the reader to consult an optometrist if the O and X disappear
d. To demonstrate that vision is a passive process

6. Based on the passage, which of the following statements is true?

a. The brain cannot accurately reflect reality
b. Glasses correct the blind spot caused by the optical nerve
c. Vision is the least important sense
d. The brain fills in gaps in the visual field

7. The author mentions the nose to illustrate what point?

a. The brain filters out some visual information
b. Not all senses work the same way
c. Perception is a passive process
d. The sense of smell filters out information

8. Which of the following statements can be inferred from the second paragraph?

a. The brain filters out the sound created by the shape of the ears
b. The brain does not perceive all activity in the visual field
c. Closing one eye affects depth perception
d. The brain evolved as a result of environmental factors

Questions 9 to 17 pertain to the following passage:

Oppositional Defiant Disorder

On a bad day, have you ever been irritable? Have you ever used a harsh tone or even been verbally disrespectful to your parents or teachers? Everyone has a short temper from time to time, but current statistics indicate that between 16% and 20% of a school's population suffer from a psychological condition known as Oppositional Defiance Disorder, or ODD.

ODD symptoms include difficulty complying with adult requests, excessive arguments with adults, temper tantrums, difficulty accepting responsibility for actions, low frustration tolerance, and behaviors intended to annoy or upset adults. Parents of children with ODD can often feel as though their whole relationship is based on conflict after conflict.

Unfortunately, ODD can be caused by a number of factors. Some students affected by ODD suffer abuse, neglect, and severe or unpredictable discipline at home. Others have parents with mood disorders or have experienced family violence. Various types of therapy are helpful in treating ODD, and some drugs can treat particular symptoms. However, no single cure exists.

The best advice from professionals is directed toward parents. Therapists encourage parents to avoid situations that usually end in power struggles, to try not to feed into oppositional behavior by reacting emotionally, to praise positive behaviors, and to discourage negative behaviors with timeouts instead of harsh discipline.

9. Which of the following statements can be inferred from paragraph 4?

a. Parents of children with ODD are bad parents
b. ODD is not a real psychological disorder
c. Medication can worsen ODD
d. Reacting emotionally to defiant behavior might worsen the behavior

10. Which of the following best describes the main idea of this passage?

a. ODD has no cause
b. ODD is a complex condition
c. Parents with ODD should seek support
d. Parents are the cause of ODD

11. As used in this passage, the word *oppositional* most nearly means:

a. Uncooperative
b. Violent
c. Passive aggressive
d. Altruistic

12. Which of the following can be inferred from paragraph one?

a. Most children who speak harshly to their parents have ODD
b. Most people exhibit symptoms of ODD occasionally
c. Between 16% and 20% of the school population has been abused
d. A short temper is a symptom of obsessive-compulsive disorder

13. As used in this passage, the phrase *feed into* most nearly means:

a. Discourage
b. Ignore
c. Encourage
d. Abuse

14. As used in this passage, the phrase *low frustration tolerance* most nearly means:

a. Patience
b. Low IQ
c. Difficulty dealing with frustration
d. The ability to cope with frustration

15. The author's purpose in writing this passage is to:

a. Express frustration about ODD
b. Prove that parents are the cause of ODD
c. Inform the reader about this complex condition
d. Persuade the reader to keep students with ODD out of public school

16. **According to the passage, which of the following is a cause of ODD?**
   a. Excessive television viewing
   b. Poor diet
   c. Severe or unpredictable punishment
   d. Low IQ

17. **Based on the passage, which of the following statements seems most true?**
   a. A variety of parenting techniques can be used to help children with ODD
   b. Children with ODD must be physically aggressive to be diagnosed
   c. Parents of children with ODD often engage in risk-taking activities
   d. Harsh disciplinary measures must be used to control children with ODD

Questions 18 to 21 pertain to the following passage:

> Protozoa are microscopic, one-celled organisms that can be free-living or parasitic in nature. They are able to multiply in humans, a factor which contributes to their survival and also permits serious infections to develop from just a single organism. Transmission of protozoa that live in the human intestine to another human typically occurs by a fecal-oral route (for example, contaminated food or water, or person-to-person contact). Protozoa that thrive in the blood or tissue of humans are transmitted to their human hosts by an arthropod vector (for example, through the bite of a mosquito or sand fly).
>
> Helminths are large, multicellular organisms that are generally visible to the naked eye in their adult stages. Like protozoa, helminths can be either free-living or parasitic in nature. In their adult form, helminths cannot multiply in humans. There are three main groups of helminths (derived from the Greek word for worms) that are human parasites:

- *Flatworms* (platyhelminths) – these include the trematodes (flukes) and cestodes (tapeworms)
- *Thorny-headed worms* (acanthocephalins) – the adult forms of these worms reside in the gastrointestinal tract. The acanthocephala are thought to be intermediate between the cestodes and nematodes
- *Roundworms* (nematodes) – the adult forms of these worms can reside in the gastrointestinal tract, blood, lymphatic system or subcutaneous tissues. Alternatively, the immature (larval) states can cause disease through their infection of various body tissues

18. **As used in this passage, the word "parasite" means:**
   a. A person who lives in Paris
   b. An organism that live on or in another organism
   c. Microscopic insects
   d. A person who takes advantage of the generosity of others

19. **According to the passage, adult Roundworms can live in:**
   a. the arthropod vector
   b. fecal matter
   c. the subcutaneous tissue of humans
   d. contaminated water

20. You can infer from this passage that:

a. larval stages of parasites are more dangerous than the adult forms
b. mosquitoes do not transmit parasites
c. worms cannot infect humans
d. clean sanitary conditions will keep you free of protozoa

21. According to the passage, which of the following is true?

I. Protozoa live in the blood or tissue of humans
II. Adult helminthes cannot reproduce in humans
III. Adult Thorny-headed worms live in the intestinal tract

a. I only
b. II only
c. I and II only
d. I, II, and III

Questions 22 to 24 pertain to the following passage:

About 17 million children and adults in the United States suffer from asthma, a condition that makes it hard to breathe. Today it is a problem that is treatable with modern medicine. In days gone by, there were many different superstitions about how to cure asthma. Some people thought that eating crickets with a little wine would help. Eating raw cat's meat might be the cure. Another idea was to try gathering some spiders' webs, rolling them into a ball, and then swallowing them. People also thought that if you ate a diet of only boiled carrots for two weeks, your asthma might go away. This carrot diet may have done some good for asthma patients since vitamin A in carrots is good for the lungs.

22. Which of the following would be a good title for the passage?

a. Asthma in the United States
b. Methods of treating asthma
c. Old wives' tales
d. Superstitions about asthma

23. The fact that 17 million children and adults in the United States suffer from asthma is probably the opening sentence of the passage because:

a. It explains why people in times gone by might have found a need to try homemade cures
b. It creates a contrast between today and the past
c. It lets the reader know that many people have asthma
d. It is a warning that anyone could get asthma

24. The main purpose of the passage is to:

a. Describe herbal remedies
b. Explain some of the measures for treating asthma from long ago
c. Define superstitions
d. Extol the virtues of modern medicine

Questions 25 and 26 pertain to the following passage:

During the last 100 years of medical science, the drugs that have been developed have altered the way people live all over the world. Over-the-counter and prescription drugs are now the key for dealing with diseases, bodily harm, and medical issues. Drugs like these are used to add longevity and quality to people's lives. But not all drugs are healthy for every person. A drug does not necessarily have to be illegal to be abused or misused. Some ways that drugs are misused include taking more or less of the drug than is needed, using a drug that is meant for another person, taking a drug for longer than needed, taking two or more drugs at a time, or using a drug for a reason that has nothing to do with being healthy. Thousands of people die from drug misuse or abuse every year in the United States.

25. According to the passage, which of the following is an example of misusing a drug?

a. Taking more of a prescription drug than the doctor ordered
b. Taking an antibiotic to kill harmful bacteria
c. Experiencing a side effect from an over-the-counter drug
d. Throwing away a medication that has passed the expiration date

26. According to the passage, which of the following is not true?

a. Over-the-counter drugs are used for medical issues
b. Every year, thousands of people in the United States die due to using drugs the wrong way
c. Medical science has come a long way in the last century
d. All drugs add longevity to a person's life

Questions 27 to 32 pertain to the following passage:

Peanut allergy is the most prevalent food allergy in the United States, affecting around one and a half million people, and it is potentially on the rise in children in the United States. While thought to be the most common cause of food-related death, deaths from food allergies are very rare. The allergy typically begins at a very young age and remains present for life for most people. Approximately one-fifth to one-quarter of children with a peanut allergy, however, outgrow it. Treatment involves careful avoidance of peanuts or any food that may contain peanut pieces or oils. For some sufferers, exposure to even the smallest amount of peanut product can trigger a serious reaction.

Symptoms of peanut allergy can include skin reactions, itching around the mouth, digestive problems, shortness of breath, and runny or stuffy nose. The most severe peanut allergies can result in anaphylaxis, which requires immediate treatment with epinephrine. Up to one-third of people with peanut allergies have severe reactions. Without treatment, anaphylactic shock can result in death due to obstruction of the airway, or heart failure. Signs of anaphylaxis include constriction of airways and difficulty breathing, shock, a rapid pulse, and dizziness or lightheadedness.

As of yet, there is no treatment to prevent or cure allergic reactions to peanuts. In May of 2008, however, Duke University Medical Center food allergy experts announced that they expect to offer a treatment for peanut allergies within five years.

Scientists do not know for sure why peanut proteins induce allergic reactions, nor do they know why some people develop peanut allergies while others do not. There is a strong genetic component to allergies: if one of a child's parents has an allergy, the child has an almost 50% chance of developing an allergy. If both parents have an allergy, the odds increase to about 70%.

Someone suffering from a peanut allergy needs to be cautious about the foods he or she eats and the products he or she puts on his or her skin. Common foods that should be checked for peanut content are ground nuts, cereals, granola, grain breads, energy bars, and salad dressings. Store prepared cookies, pastries, and frozen desserts like ice cream can also contain peanuts. Additionally, many cuisines use peanuts in cooking – watch for peanut content in African, Chinese, Indonesian, Mexican, Thai, and Vietnamese dishes.

Parents of children with peanut allergies should notify key people (child care providers, school personnel, etc.) that their child has a peanut allergy, explain peanut allergy symptoms to them, make sure that the child's epinephrine auto injector is always available, write an action plan of care for their child when he or she has an allergic reaction to peanuts, have their child wear a medical alert bracelet or necklace, and discourage their child from sharing foods.

27. According to the passage, approximately what percentage of people with peanut allergies have severe reactions?

a. Up to 11%
b. Up to 22%
c. Up to 33%
d. Up to 55%

28. By what date do Duke University allergy experts expect to offer a treatment for peanut allergies?

a. 2008
b. 2009
c. 2010
d. 2013

29. Which of the following is not a type of cuisine the passage suggests often contains peanuts?

a. African
b. Italian
c. Vietnamese
d. Mexican

30. Which allergy does the article state is thought to be the most common cause of food-related death?

a. Peanut
b. Tree nut
c. Bee sting
d. Poison oak

31. It can be inferred from the passage that children with peanut allergies should be discouraged from sharing food because:

a. Peanut allergies can be contagious
b. People suffering from peanut allergies are more susceptible to bad hygiene
c. Many foods contain peanut content and it is important to be very careful when you don't know what you're eating
d. Scientists don't know why some people develop peanut allergies

32. Which of the following does the passage not state is a sign of anaphylaxis?

a. Constriction of airways
b. Shock
c. A rapid pulse
d. Running or stuffy nose

Questions 33 to 36 pertain to the following passage:

> Among the Atkins, South Beach and other diets people embark upon for health and weight loss is the so-called Paleolithic Diet in which adherents eat what they believe to be a diet similar to that consumed by humans during the Paleolithic era. The diet consists of food that can be hunted or gathered: primarily of meat, fish, vegetables, fruits, roots, and nuts. It does not allow for grains, legumes, dairy, salt, refined sugars or processed oils. The idea behind the diet is that humans are genetically adapted to the diet of our Paleolithic forebears. Some studies support the idea of positive health outcomes from such a diet.

33. Which of the following does the passage not give as the name of a diet?

a. South Beach
b. Hunter Gatherer
c. Paleolithic
d. Atkins

34. Which of the following is not permitted on the Paleolithic Diet?

a. Meat
b. Dairy
c. Vegetables
d. Nuts

35. What does the passage say is the idea behind the diet?

a. That humans are genetically adapted to the diet of our Paleolithic forebears
b. That it increases health
c. That it supports weight loss
d. That it consists of food that can be hunted or gathered

36. Which of the following does the passage suggest is true?

a. No studies support the claim that the Paleolithic Diet promotes health
b. Some studies support the claim that the Paleolithic Diet promotes health
c. All studies support the claim that the Paleolithic Diet promotes health
d. No studies have been done on whether the Paleolithic Diet promotes health

Questions 37-41 refer to the following medication directions:

Directions: For the relief of headaches. Take one pill every 4 to 6 hours, not exceeding 4 in a 24-hour period. If stomach upset occurs, take with food. If pain persists more than 24 hours, contact a physician.

37. The medication should be taken:

a. 6 times a day
b. Every thirty minutes
c. On an empty stomach
d. To treat a headache

38. In the context of the passage, *upset* most nearly means:

a. Angry
b. Annoyed
c. Physical disorder
d. Confusion

39. If someone follows the directions, what is the maximum number of pills he or she should have taken before he or she should contact a physician?

a. 2
b. 3
c. 4
d. 6

40. In the context of the passage, *persists* most nearly means:

a. Tries
b. Continues
c. Hurts
d. Worsens

41. According to the instructions, what is the maximum number of pills one should take, including the first one, during the first 12 hours of using this medication?

a. 2
b. 3
c. 4
d. 5

Questions 42-47 refer to the following medication directions:

Tips for Eating Calcium Rich Foods

- Include milk as a beverage at meals. Choose fat-free or low-fat milk.
- If you usually drink whole milk, switch gradually to fat-free milk to lower saturated fat and calories. Try reduced fat (2%), then low-fat (1%), and finally fat-free (skim).
- If you drink cappuccinos or lattes—ask for them with fat-free (skim) milk.
- Add fat-free or low-fat milk instead of water to oatmeal and hot cereals
- Use fat-free or low-fat milk when making condensed cream soups (such as cream of tomato).
- Have fat-free or low-fat yogurt as a snack.

- Make a dip for fruits or vegetables from yogurt.
- Make fruit-yogurt smoothies in the blender.
- For dessert, make chocolate or butterscotch pudding with fat-free or low-fat milk.
- Top cut-up fruit with flavored yogurt for a quick dessert.
- Top casseroles, soups, stews, or vegetables with shredded low-fat cheese.
- Top a baked potato with fat-free or low-fat yogurt.

For those who choose not to consume milk products:

- If you avoid milk because of lactose intolerance, the most reliable way to get the health benefits of milk is to choose lactose-free alternatives within the milk group, such as cheese, yogurt, or lactose-free milk, or to consume the enzyme lactase before consuming milk products.
- Calcium choices for those who do not consume milk products include:
    - Calcium fortified juices, cereals, breads, soy beverages, or rice beverages
    - Canned fish (sardines, salmon with bones) soybeans and other soy products, some other dried beans, and some leafy greens.

42. According to the passage, how can you lower saturated fat and calories in your diet?

a. Add fat-free milk to oatmeal instead of water
b. Switch to fat-free milk
c. Drink calcium-fortified juice
d. Make yogurt dip

43. What device does the author use to organize the passage?

a. Lists
b. Captions
c. Diagrams
d. Labels

44. How much fat does reduced fat milk contain?

a. 0 percent
b. 1 percent
c. 2 percent
d. 3 percent

45. Which of the following is true about calcium rich foods?

I. Canned salmon with bones contains calcium
II. Cheese is a lactose-free food
III. Condensed soup made with water is a calcium rich food

a. I only
b. I and II only
c. II and III only
d. III only

46. What information should the author include to help clarify information in the passage?

a. The fat content of yogurt
b. How much calcium is in fortified juice
c. Which leafy greens contain calcium
d. The definition of lactose intolerance

47. The style of this passage is most like that found in a(n):

a. Tourist guidebook
b. Informal letter
c. Encyclopedia
d. Health textbook

Vocabulary and General Knowledge

48. What is the best definition for the word *latent*?

a. Thorough
b. Dormant
c. Current
d. Obvious

49. What is the meaning of the word *derelict*?

a. Tentative
b. Redundant
c. Revived
d. Dilapidated

50. What is the best definition of the word *aversion*?

a. attraction
b. antithesis
c. abhorrence
d. adequate

51. What is the meaning of the word *diffuse*?

a. Disseminate
b. Compress
c. Distinct
d. Widen

52. What is the meaning of the word *anterior*?

a. Previous
b. Front
c. Crucial
d. Final

53. What is the meaning of the word *rescinded*?

a. Restored
b. Denied
c. Acquired
d. Revoked

54. What is the best definition for the word *comply*?

a. Follow
b. Affect
c. Depend
d. Decline

55. Select the meaning of the underlined word in this sentence:

Despite the leadership problems that plagued the corporation, the CEO was quick to assert his authority to ensure that business continued as usual.

a. Maintain
b. Prevent
c. Censure
d. Accept

56. What is the meaning of the word *occlude*?

a. Release
b. Invade
c. Prevent
d. Direct

57. Select the meaning of the underlined word in this sentence:

Having spent hours preparing her research, Eirinn felt that her colleague's hasty rejection of her presentation was untoward and merited a formal complaint.

a. Inappropriate
b. Delicate
c. Friendly
d. Eager

58. What is the best definition for the word *superficial*?

a. Surface
b. Backward
c. Awkward
d. Intense

59. What is the best definition for the word *inverted*?

a. Credible
b. Benign
c. Forward
d. Reversed

60. What is the meaning of the word *void*?

a. Emit
b. Determine
c. Confirm
d. Prevent

61. Select the meaning of the underlined word in this sentence:

Fearful that the fever might have an adverse effect, Catriona called the doctor for an emergency appointment.

a. Preventive
b. Auspicious
c. Negative
d. Reckless

62. What is the meaning of the word *contingent*?

a. Dependent
b. Protective
c. Definite
d. Intended

63. Select the meaning of the underlined word in this sentence:

Philippa was upset about the doctor's unwillingness to release her from the hospital for another week, so she demanded that he explain his <u>rationale</u> to her.

a. Description
b. Justification
c. Persistence
d. Ambiguity

64. What is the best definition for the word *patent*?

a. Inconspicuous
b. Privileged
c. Careless
d. Unconcealed

65. What is the best definition for the word *labile*?

a. External
b. Meticulous
c. Fluctuating
d. Integral

66. What is the best definition for the word *impending*?

a. Demanding
b. Approaching
c. Perilous
d. Producing

67. What is the meaning of the word *cacophony*?

a. Din
b. Dialogue
c. Divination
d. Diversity

68. What is the meaning of the word *boisterous*?

a. Obnoxious
b. Exuberant
c. Masculine
d. Robust

69. Select the meaning of the underlined word in this sentence:

The meeting fell into an uncomfortable silence after Bosworth's acerbic comment on the new CEO's weight.

a. Uncontrolled
b. Solicitous
c. Untruthful
d. Scathing

70. What is the best definition for the word *cloistered*?

a. Sweetened
b. Dampened
c. Deafened
d. Sheltered

71. What is the best definition for the word *adsorb*?

a. Divide
b. Process
c. Accumulate
d. Contain

72. What is the best definition for the word *compensatory*?

a. Corrupted
b. Offsetting
c. Varying
d. Contradictory

73. What is the meaning of the word *incompatible*?

a. Conflicting
b. Subsequent
c. Relevant
d. Suitable

74. What is the best definition for the word *lateral*?

a. Positive
b. Central
c. Sideward
d. Serious

75. What is the meaning of the word *vivacious*?

a. Viral
b. Vindictive
c. Vitriolic
d. Vigorous

76. What is the meaning of the word *exiguous*?

a. Superfluous
b. Defective
c. Inadequate
d. Eager

77. What is the meaning of the word *untenable*?

a. Logical
b. Groundless
c. Opaque
d. Analogous

78. What is the best definition for the word *placate*?

a. Authorize
b. Incite
c. Clarify
d. Comfort

79. What is the best definition for the word *inure*?

a. Toughen
b. Pretend
c. Anticipate
d. Forget

80. What is the best definition for the word *clement*?

a. Difficult
b. Angry
c. Favorable
d. Righteous

81. What is the meaning of the word *malign*?

a. Harm
b. Submit
c. Improve
d. Conceive

82. What is the best definition for the word *synergy*?

a. Delay
b. Harmony
c. Distress
d. Hindrance

83. What is the best definition for the word *recede*?

a. Increase
b. Dilate
c. Present
d. Retreat

84. What is the best definition for the word *inflame*?

a. Worsen
b. Ignite
c. Lull
d. Endanger

85. What is the meaning of the word *detriment*?

a. Drawback
b. Retribution
c. Excitement
d. Indulgence

86. What is the meaning of the word *turgid*?

a. Intricate
b. Murky
c. Inflated
d. Acceptable

87. What is the meaning of the word *paucity*?

a. Hunger
b. Affluence
c. Lack
d. Insistence

88. What is the best definition for the word *tractable*?

a. Interactive
b. Irresistible
c. Alluring
d. Amenable

89. What is the meaning of the word *austere*?

a. Calm
b. Stark
c. Dependable
d. Greedy

90. What is the best definition for the word *delineate*?

a. Open
b. Confuse
c. Brag
d. Detail

91. What is the best definition for the word *expedient*?

a. Grateful
b. Practical
c. Unprofitable
d. Substitute

92. What is the meaning of the word *facilitate*?

a. recast
b. smooth
c. thwart
d. decide

93. What is the meaning of the word *restive*?

a. Frightened
b. Hostile
c. Tense
d. Apathetic

94. What is the best definition for the word *recourse*?

a. Ambush
b. Obligation
c. Option
d. Proposal

95. What is the best definition for the word *impetus*?

a. Motivation
b. Diversion
c. Authority
d. Prevention

96. What is the best definition for the word *salient*?

a. Acceptable
b. Ordinary
c. Peripheral
d. Important

97. What is the meaning of the word *laconic*?

a. Slow
b. Incomplete
c. Brief
d. Tidy

Grammar

98. Select the word that makes this sentence grammatically correct:

Writing, doing yoga, and ________ were her favorite activities.

a. playing volleyball
b. doing volleyball
c. making volleyball
d. volleyballing

99. Select the word that makes this sentence grammatically correct:

Every kid in the neighborhood has ______ own bicycle.

a. its
b. him
c. our
d. her

100. Select the phrase that makes this sentence grammatically correct:

Maria thinks it is unfair that she has to ______ with her younger brother's whining all the time.

a. put up
b. put down
c. put in
d. put off

101. Select the word that makes this sentence grammatically correct:

Enrique will ______ harder as the date of the test draws nearer.

a. studying
b. have studied
c. studyed
d. study

102. Select the word that makes this sentence grammatically correct:

Suzanna replied ________ to her sister's plea to help her with her finances.

a. hasty
b. sympathetically
c. generous
d. friendly

103. Select the word that makes this sentence grammatically correct:

A team of scientists _______ studying a new species of frog.

a. is
b. are
c. were
d. have

104. Select the word that makes this sentence grammatically correct:

Everyone we invited to the party ________, so it was a huge success!

a. shown up
b. showed up
c. showed upped
d. shows up

105. Which word is not spelled correctly in the context of the following sentence?

Buying prescents for others is not the most authentic way to develop new friendships.

a. buying
b. prescents
c. authentic
d. friendships

106. Which word is not spelled correctly in the context of the following sentence?

Raymond feels children misbehave too much, that parents have lost their athority, and that they need to emphasize discipline more.

a. misbehave
b. emphasize
c. discipline
d. athority

107. Select the word that makes this sentence grammatically correct:

Each received ______ trophy to take home.

a. it's
b. her
c. their
d. our

108. Select the word that makes this sentence grammatically correct:

Eli ________ insisted that it wasn't his fault.

a. tearfully
b. adamant
c. emphatic
d. joyful

109. Select the word that makes this sentence grammatically correct:

Margaret ________ the committee into thinking the project was all her work.

a. missled
b. misled
c. mislead
d. mislled

110. Select the word that makes this sentence grammatically correct:

Tomorrow, Atticus will ________ cupcakes to school.

a. brought
b. had brought
c. bring
d. broughten

111. Select the word that makes this sentence grammatically correct:

Each participant in the course on being a good father received ________ own signed copy of the teacher's book.

a. their
b. our
c. his
d. ones

112. Select the word that makes this sentence grammatically correct:

Several of the runners __________ not to complete the race; they met the rest of us by the finish line.

a. decide
b. decided
c. decides
d. were deciding

113. Select the word that makes this sentence grammatically correct:

Stephanie writes _________.

a. good
b. well
c. clear
d. articulate

114. Which word is not spelled correctly in the context of the following sentence?

Judy's neighbor was friends with her neice and invited her on the holiday sleigh ride.

a. Neighbor
b. Friends
c. Neice
d. Sleigh

115. Which word is not spelled correctly in the context of the following sentence?

Oscar was truely sad to be enforcing the hateful judgment.

a. truely
b. enforcing
c. hateful
d. judgment

116. Select the word or phrase that makes the following sentence grammatically correct.

Everyone who visits the fine art museum ________ to see the new Manet exhibit.

a. should
b. needs
c. have
d. must

117. Select the word or phrase that makes the following sentence grammatically correct.

Their experience at the opera, viewing the company's production of Turandot, was so bad that _______ have not yet returned.

a. he and she
b. we
c. him and her
d. him and I

118. Select the word or phrase that makes the following sentence grammatically correct.

After hearing about everyone's positive experience at the party, Desmond realized that he __________.

a. should have went
b. should have gone
c. should go
d. should have been

119. Select the word or phrase that makes the following sentence grammatically correct.

Loman made a quick telephone call to the person ______ was responsible for organizing the event.

a. that
b. which
c. who
d. this

120. Select the word or phrase that makes the following sentence grammatically correct.

Nessa returned the lost cat to the Millers after seeing the sign and realizing that the cat was ________.

a. hers
b. his
c. ours
d. theirs

121. Select the word or phrase that makes the following sentence grammatically correct.

See to it that Derek or Una ________ the box of clothing that is to be donated to the church rummage sale.

a. are collecting
b. collects
c. collect
d. would collect

122. Select the word or phrase that makes the following sentence grammatically correct.

Neither Jane nor ________ knows at what time the surprise party for Richard is supposed to begin.

a. she
b. him
c. me
d. they

123. Select the word or phrase that makes the following sentence grammatically correct.

Ieva pointed a quivering finger at the butler and exclaimed, "It was ________! He stole the pearls from my room."

a. him
b. his
c. himself
d. he

124. Select the word or phrase that makes the following sentence grammatically correct.

The grand prize of $10,000 will be given to ________ arrives at the finish line first.

a. who
b. whom
c. whoever
d. whomever

125. Select the word or phrase that makes the following sentence grammatically correct.

Angus knew his mobile phone was gone for good when he realized that he had forgotten to take it ________ the roof of the car before he started driving.

a. off
b. off of
c. off from
d. away from

126. Select the word or phrase that makes the following sentence grammatically correct.

The committee ________ in disagreement about the decorations for the upcoming event.

a. is
b. were
c. was
d. would be

127. Select the word or phrase that makes the following sentence grammatically correct.

About three o'clock in the afternoon, a parched Veronika realized that she had not ________ any water all day.

a. drank
b. drunk
c. drink
d. drunken

128. Select the word or phrase that makes the following sentence grammatically correct.

The priest quoted I Corinthians 2.9: "What no eye has _______, what no ear has heard, and what no human mind has conceived..."

a. saw
b. see
c. seeing
d. seen

129. Select the word or phrase that makes the following sentence grammatically correct.

When the ice-cream man arrives later today, the children _______________.

a. were excited
b. would be excited
c. will be excited
d. would have been excited

130. Select the word or phrase that makes the following sentence grammatically correct.

Once I complete this final pose, I ______________ yoga for two full hours.

a. will have been doing
b. will do
c. will be doing
d. would be doing

131. Select the word or phrase that makes the following sentence grammatically correct.

Effie contacted a travel agent to help her find the vacation plan _________ offered her the best options.

a. that
b. than
c. which
d. who

132. Select the word or phrase that makes the following sentence grammatically correct.

Aidan performed the solo __________, far worse than anyone had expected.

a. real bad
b. real badly
c. really bad
d. really badly

133. Select the word or phrase that makes the following sentence grammatically correct.

Grant demanded of his teenage son, "_____________________?"

a. Where did you go to
b. Where did you go from
c. Where did you go at
d. Where did you go

134. Select the word or phrase that makes the following sentence grammatically correct.

I should _________ attended the concert, since everyone mentioned how fun it was.

a. of
b. be
c. have
d. has

135. Select the punctuation that makes the following sentence grammatically correct.

When Finn called his mother he did not tell her about all of his plans.

a. mother, he
b. Finn, called
c. not, tell
d. when, Finn

136. Select the word or phrase that makes the following sentence grammatically correct.

Professor Howard had thirty-five students in the class, and she stayed up late grading all the _________ papers.

a. student's
b. students
c. students's
d. students'

137. Select the word or phrase that makes the following sentence grammatically correct.

The kindergarten teacher praised Kama after she did _______ on the assignment.

a. good
b. great
c. worse
d. well

138. Select the punctuation that makes the following sentence grammatically correct.

Olaf planned to see the movie but he could not go after he caught the flu.

a. but, he
b. movie, he
c. movie, but
d. but; he

139. Select the word or phrase that makes the following sentence grammatically correct.

Maura knocked on the door of _______________ dorm room.

a. Melissa and Caroline's
b. Melissa's and Caroline
c. Melissa's and Caroline's
d. Melissa and Caroline

140. Select the expression that uses the correct punctuation to complete the following sentence.

Doctor Marshall has had his medical license since the early __________.

a. 1980's
b. 1980s'
c. 1980s
d. '1980s

141. Select the word or phrase that makes the following sentence grammatically correct.

Jean intended to hold the picnic on Saturday, ________ the sudden deluge forced her to reschedule it.

a. and
b. however
c. but
d. or

142. Select the word or phrase that makes the following sentence grammatically correct.

The professor announced to the class, "To prevent the temptation for cheating, I will collect your study notes ________ the exam."

a. during
b. before
c. upon
d. after

143. Select the combination of words that makes the following sentence grammatically correct.

I want to _________ a change in the program, so I will have to present a solution that will have a strong ________ on the board.

a. affect, affect
b. affect, effect
c. effect, effect
d. effect, affect

144. Select the combination of words that makes the following sentence grammatically correct.

Due to company policy, Eleanora could not ________ any gifts ___________ from other company employees, and only on her birthday.

a. accept, except
b. accept, accept
c. except, accept
d. except, except

145. Select the combination of words that makes the following sentence grammatically correct.

To __________ that you are properly covered, be sure to __________ your home against fire.

a. ensure, ensure
b. insure, insure
c. insure, ensure
d. ensure, insure

146. Disney films often use the same voice actors; _______, Sterling Holloway was the voice for Winnie the Pooh, the stork in Dumbo, the snake Kaa in Jungle Book, and the Cheshire Cat in Alice in Wonderland.

a. but
b. for instance
c. thus
d. so

147. Choose the word or words that best fill the blank.

Many similarities exist between the film Star Wars IV: A New Hope and a Japanese film called The Hidden Fortress, _______ , Star Wars director George Lucas openly acknowledges the film as a significant influence.

a. however
b. or
c. in fact
d. yet

Mathematics

148. What number is 25% of 400?

a. 100
b. 200
c. 800
d. 10,000

149. What is the reciprocal of 6?

a. $\frac{1}{2}$
b. $\frac{1}{3}$
c. $\frac{1}{6}$
d. $\frac{1}{12}$

150. A roast was cooked at 325 °F in the oven for 4 hours. The internal temperature of the roast rose from 32 °F to 145 °F. What was the average rise in temperature per hour?

a. 20.2 °F/hr
b. 28.25 °F/hr
c. 32.03 °F/hr
d. 37 °F/hr

151. Your supervisor instructs you to purchase 240 pens and 6 staplers for the nurse's station. Pens are purchase in sets of 6 for $2.35 per pack. Staplers are sold in sets of 2 for $12.95 per set. How much will purchasing these products cost?

a. $132.85
b. $145.75
c. $162.90
d. $225.05

152. Which of the following percentages is equivalent to the decimal 0.45?

a. 0.045%
b. 0.45%
c. 4.5%
d. 45%

153. A vitamin's expiration date has passed. It was supposed to contain 500 mg of calcium, but it has lost 325 mg of calcium. How many mg of calcium remain?

a. 135 mg
b. 175 mg
c. 185 mg
d. 200 mg

154. You have orders to give a patient 20 mg of a certain substance. The concentration of the substance within the medication is 4 mg per 5-mL dose. How much medication should be given?

a. 15 mL
b. 20 mL
c. 25 mL
d. 30 mL

155. In the number 743.25 which digit represents the tenths space?

a. 2
b. 3
c. 4
d. 5

156. Which of these percentages is equivalent to the decimal 1.25?

a. 0.125%
b. 12.5%
c. 125%
d. 1250%

157. If the average person drinks eight 8-oz glasses of water per day, a person who drinks 12.8 oz of water after a morning exercise session has consumed what fraction of the daily average?

a. 1/3
b. 1/5
c. 1/7
d. 1/9

158. What number is 33% of 300?

a. 3
b. 9
c. 33
d. 99

159. You need $\frac{4}{5}$ cup of water for a recipe. You accidentally put $\frac{1}{3}$ cup into the mixing bowl with the dry ingredients. How much more water do you need to add?

a. $\frac{1}{3}$ cups
b. $\frac{2}{3}$ cups
c. $\frac{1}{15}$ cups
d. $\frac{7}{15}$ cups

160. $\frac{3}{4} - \frac{1}{2} = ?$

a. $\frac{1}{4}$
b. $\frac{1}{3}$
c. $\frac{1}{2}$
d. $\frac{2}{3}$

161. In your class there are 48 students, 32 of whom are female. Approximately what percentage of the class is male?

a. 25%
b. 33%
c. 45%
d. 66%

162. Fried's rule for computing an infant's dose of medication is:

$$\text{infant's dose} = \frac{[\text{child's age in months}] \times [\text{adult dose}]}{150}$$

If the adult dose of medication is 15 mg, how much should be given to a 2-year-old child?

a. 1.2 mg
b. 2.4 mg
c. 3.6 mg
d. 4.8 mg

163. $7\frac{1}{2} - 5\frac{3}{8} = ?$

a. $1\frac{1}{2}$
b. $1\frac{2}{3}$
c. $2\frac{1}{8}$
d. $3\frac{1}{4}$

164. 35 is 20% of what number?

a. 175
b. 186
c. 190
d. 220

165. $6 \times 0 \times 5 = ?$

a. 30
b. 11
c. 25
d. 0

166. $\mathbf{7.95 \div 1.5} = ?$

a. 2.4
b. 5.3
c. 6.2
d. 7.3

167. The fraction $\frac{7}{10}$ is equivalent to which decimal?

a. 0.007
b. 0.07
c. 0.7
d. 7.10

168. The fraction $\frac{4}{8}$ is equivalent to which decimal?

a. 0.05
b. 0.48
c. 0.5
d. 4.8

169. $\mathbf{-32 + 7} = ?$

a. –25
b. 25
c. –26
d. 26

170. The percentage 41% is equivalent to which decimal?

a. 4.1
b. 0.41
c. 0.041
d. 0.0041

171. $\mathbf{248 + 311} = ?$

a. 557
b. 559
c. 659
d. 667

172. $\mathbf{13,980 + 7,031} = ?$

a. 20,010
b. 20.911
c. 21,011
d. 21,911

173. $\mathbf{8,537 - 6,316} = ?$

a. 1,221
b. 2,221
c. 2,243
d. 2,841

174. $\mathbf{643 \times 72} = ?$

a. 44,096
b. 44,186
c. 46,296
d. 45,576

175. $\mathbf{18,144 \div 63} = ?$

a. 256
b. 258
c. 286
d. 288

176. $\mathbf{3.5 + 10.3 + 0.63} = ?$

a. 11.28
b. 13.58
c. 14.43
d. 20.10

177. $\mathbf{0.19 \times 0.23} = ?$

a. 0.3470
b. 0.4370
c. 0.0347
d. 0.0437

178. The fraction $\frac{0.3}{0.08}$ is equal to which decimal?

a. 0.0375
b. 0.375
c. 3.75
d. 37.5

179. Which numeral is in the thousandths place in 0.5643?

a. 5
b. 6
c. 4
d. 3

180. $\mathbf{0.43 - 0.17} = ?$

a. 0.26
b. 2.6
c. 0.36
d. 3.6

181. Round this decimal to the nearest hundredth: 0.3489

a. 0.33
b. 0.349
c. 0.348
d. 0.35

182. $\mathbf{2\frac{1}{2} + 3 + \frac{1}{7}} = ?$

a. $5\frac{9}{14}$
b. $6\frac{1}{2}$
c. $5\frac{5}{14}$
d. $6\frac{5}{7}$

183. $\mathbf{3\frac{1}{9} - 1\frac{1}{4}} = ?$

a. $1\frac{5}{6}$
b. $1\frac{31}{36}$
c. $2\frac{5}{36}$
d. $2\frac{31}{36}$

184. $\mathbf{3\frac{1}{8} \times 6\frac{1}{3} \times 2\frac{2}{5}} = ?$

a. $47\frac{1}{2}$
b. $36\frac{7}{8}$
c. $40\frac{3}{8}$
d. $42\frac{4}{5}$

185. $\mathbf{\frac{1}{8} \div \frac{4}{5}} = ?$

a. $\frac{5}{32}$
b. $\frac{1}{10}$
c. $\frac{2}{5}$
d. $\frac{3}{8}$

186. Solve for *n* in the following equation:

$$\frac{n}{5} = \frac{12}{20}$$

a. 2
b. 3
c. 4
d. 5

187. Reduce $\mathbf{\frac{17}{102}}$ to the lowest possible terms.

a. $\frac{1}{4}$
b. $\frac{5}{6}$
c. $\frac{1}{6}$
d. $\frac{3}{4}$

188. Express $\frac{99}{14}$ as a mixed number.

a. $7\frac{1}{14}$
b. $7\frac{3}{14}$
c. $7\frac{11}{14}$
d. $7\frac{5}{14}$

189. The number 3 is what percentage of 50?

a. 3%
b. 4%
c. 5%
d. 6%

190. Three fifths of 60 equals:

a. 30
b. 32
c. 36
d. 40

191. What number is 0.5% of 40?

a. 0.2
b. 0.8
c. 2.0
d. 8.0

192. What percentage is equivalent to a 2:10 ratio?

a. 2%
b. 3%
c. 5%
d. 20%

193. What percentage is equivalent to the fraction $\frac{3}{5}$?

a. 40%
b. 4%
c. 60%
d. 6%

194. Which of the following fractions represents the most simplified form of the percentage 15%?

a. $\frac{3}{20}$
b. $\frac{15}{100}$
c. $\frac{5}{20}$
d. $\frac{20}{3}$

195. 1.5 is 1.25% of what number?

a. 80
b. 120
c. 140
d. 150

196. 8 is 25% of what number?

a. 16
b. 24
c. 32
d. 40

197. 18 is 40% of what number?

a. 36
b. 360
c. 45
d. 450

Biology

198. Which of the following sentences is true?

a. All organisms begin life as a single cell
b. All organisms begin life as multi-cellular
c. Some organisms begin life as a single cell and others as multi-cellular
d. None of the above

199. Which of the following is the best definition for metabolism?

a. The process by which organisms lose weight
b. The process by which organisms use energy
c. The process by which organisms return to homeostasis
d. The process by which organisms leave homeostasis

200. Which of the following is not true for all cells?

a. Cells are the basic structures of any organism
b. Cells can only reproduce from existing cells
c. Cells are the smallest unit of any life form that carries the information needed for all life processes
d. All cells are also called eukaryotes

201. What are the two types of cellular transport?

a. Passive and diffusion
b. Diffusion and active
c. Active and passive
d. Kinetic and active

202. What does <u>aerobic</u> mean?

a. In the presence of oxygen
b. Calorie-burning
c. Heated
d. Anabolic

203. When both parents give offspring the same allele, the offspring is ______ for that trait.

a. Heterozygous
b. Homozygous
c. Recessive
d. Dominant

204. Genetics is the study of:

a. Anatomy
b. Physiology
c. Heredity
d. Science

205. Scientists suggest that ______ has occurred through a process called ______.

a. evolution… differentiation
b. evolution… natural selection
c. natural selection… homeostasis
d. homeostasis… reproduction

206. Which of the following correctly lists the cellular hierarchy from the simplest to the most complex structure?

a. tissue, cell, organ, organ system, organism
b. organism, organ system, organ, tissue, cell
c. organ system, organism, organ, tissue, cell
d. cell, tissue, organ, organ system, organism

207. If a cell is placed in a hypertonic solution, what will happen to the cell?

a. It will swell
b. It will shrink
c. It will stay the same
d. It does not affect the cell

208. What is the longest phase of the cell cycle?

a. mitosis
b. cytokinesis
c. interphase
d. metaphase

Use the following Punnett Square to answer questions 209 and 210:

B = alleles for brown eyes; g = alleles for green eyes

	B	**g**
B	BB	Bg
g	Bg	gg

209. Which word describes the allele for green eyes?

a. dominant
b. recessive
c. homozygous
d. heterozygous

210. What is the possibility that the offspring produced will have brown eyes?

a. 25%
b. 50%
c. 75%
d. 100%

211. Which of the following correctly describes the trait Ll, if "L" represents tallness and "l" represents shortness?

a. heterozygous genotype and tall phenotype
b. heterozygous phenotype and tall genotype
c. homozygous genotype and short phenotype
d. homozygous phenotype and short genotype

212. Which of the following is an example of a non-communicable disease?

a. influenza
b. tuberculosis
c. arthritis
d. measles

213. All living organisms on Earth utilize:

a. Oxygen
b. Light
c. Sexual reproduction
d. A triplet genetic code

214. Which of the following is not a nitrogenous base found in DNA?

a. Thymine
b. Uracil
c. Guanine
d. Adenine

215. Which of the following is true?

a. The basic formula for a carbohydrate is $(CH_2O)_N$
b. Water bonds well with nonpolar substances
c. Enzymes are an example of secondary proteins
d. An exergonic reaction is one that uses up energy

216. Which cell structure is responsible for modifying substances and distributing them to their proper place in the cell?

a. Endoplasmic reticulum
b. Ribosome
c. Golgi apparatus
d. Lysosome

217. Prokaryotes do not contain:

a. cell membrane
b. cell wall
c. nucleus
d. ribosomes

218. Which stage of mitosis is occurring when the centromeres are lining up in the middle of the cell and preparing for division?

a. Metaphase
b. Anaphase
c. Prophase
d. Telophase

219. During the S phase in the Interphase stage of mitosis, what event is occurring?

a. Resting before the next cell division
b. Rapid DNA replication
c. Cytokinesis
d. Construction of microtubules which will eventually form the cytoskeleton

220. Which of the following is true of meiosis?

a. Two identical daughter cells are formed
b. It is used to replicate body cells
c. Four diploid cells are formed during Meiosis II
d. Gametes are haploid cells

221. Which of the following statements about the Krebs cycle is true?

a. It occurs only once per glucose molecule
b. It is an anaerobic process
c. It takes place in the cytoplasm
d. It starts with the conversion of one pyruvate molecule into 2 acetyl-CoA molecules

222. How is the most amount of energy released from ATP?

a. When the entire molecule of ATP has been broken apart
b. When ADP binds to another phosphate group to form ATP
c. When one phosphate group breaks off ATP to form ADP and free phosphate
d. Each time an additional phosphate group bonds with adenosine, forming ADP and then ATP

Chemistry

223. Which of the following is true?

a. Mass and weight are the same thing
b. Mass is the quantity of matter an object has
c. Mass equals twice the weight of an object
d. Mass equals half the weight of an object

224. Which of the following is not a state of matter?

a. Gas
b. Liquid
c. Lattice
d. Solid

225. What is the name for substances that cannot be broken down into simpler types of matter?

a. Electron
b. Molecules
c. Nuclei
d. Elements

226. What are the two types of measurement important in science?

a. quantitative and numerical
b. qualitative and descriptive
c. numerical and scientific
d. quantitative and qualitative

227. What is the typical way a solid would turn to a liquid and then to a gas?

a. Vaporization then melting
b. Melting then freezing
c. Vaporization then freezing
d. Melting then vaporization

228. An atom with an electrical charge is called a(n):

a. Electron
b. Ion
c. Molecule
d. Enzyme

229. When atoms of one element are combined with atoms of another element, the result is a(n) ________ of a compound.

a. Electron
b. Ion
c. Molecule
d. Enzyme

230. What is freezing point?

a. The point at which a liquid changes to a solid
b. The point at which a gas changes to a liquid
c. The point at which a gas changes to a solid
d. The point at which a liquid changes to a gas

231. The rate of a chemical reaction depends on all of the following except:

a. temperature
b. surface area
c. presence of catalysts
d. amount of mass lost

232. Which of the answer choices provided best defines the following statement:

For a given mass and constant temperature, an inverse relationship exists between the volume and pressure of a gas?

a. Ideal Gas Law
b. Boyle's Law
c. Charles' Law
d. Stefan-Boltzmann Law

233. Which of the following is exchanged between two or more atoms that undergo ionic bonding?

a. neutrons
b. transitory electrons
c. valence electrons
d. electrical charges

234. Which of the following statements is *not* true of most metals?

a. They are good conductors of heat
b. They are gases at room temperature
c. They are ductile
d. They make up the majority of elements on the periodic table

235. What is most likely the pH of a solution containing many hydroxide ions (OH^-) and few hydrogen ions (H^+)?

a. 2
b. 6
c. 7
d. 9

236. Which of the following cannot be found on the periodic table?

a. bromine
b. magnesium oxide
c. phosphorous
d. chlorine

237. Nora makes soup by adding some spices to a pot of boiling water and stirring the spices until completely dissolved. Next, she adds several chopped vegetables. What is the solute in her mixture?

a. water
b. vegetables
c. spices
d. heat

238. What law describes the electric force between two charged particles?

a. Ohm's law
b. Coulomb's law
c. The Doppler effect
d. Kirchhoff's current law

239. What process transfers thermal energy through matter directly from particle to particle?

a. convection
b. radiation
c. conduction
d. insulation

240. Which state of matter contains the least amount of kinetic energy?

a. solid
b. liquid
c. gas
d. plasma

241. Which of the following is a vector quantity?

a. Distance
b. Speed
c. Velocity
d. Time

242. As you move from left to right across the periodic table, which of the following is true?

a. Atomic radius increases
b. Electronegativity increases
c. Ionization energy decreases
d. Electron affinity decreases

243. What is the correct molecular formula for aluminum hydroxide?

a. $Al(OH)_3$
b. $AlOH_3$
c. Al_3OH
d. AlO_3H

244. According to Charles' law:

a. PV = nRT
b. temperature and volume are directly related
c. the volume of a gas is inversely related to the number of moles in that gas
d. pressure and volume of a gas are inversely related

245. What type of substance has some properties of a metal, but is made up of a mixture of different elements?

a. Metals
b. Nonmetals
c. Alloy
d. Network solids

246. The process of sublimation occurs when a ______ changes into a ________.

a. solid, gas
b. liquid, gas
c. gas, solid
d. liquid, solid

247. Decreasing a liquid's pH from 5 to 4 will increase the hydrogen ion concentration by a factor of:

a. 10
b. 100
c. 1,000
d. 10,000

Anatomy and Physiology

248.Which hormone is *not* secreted by a gland in the brain?

a. Human chorionic gonadotropin (HCG)
b. Gonadotropin releasing hormone (GnRH)
c. Luteinizing hormone (LH)
d. Follicle stimulating hormone (FSH)

249. Select the most accurate statement among the following regarding the human circulatory system:

a. All arteries carry oxygenated blood away from the heart
b. Blood flows faster through capillaries than through veins
c. The walls of both arteries and veins are made of three main layers
d. An increase in heart rate correlates with an increase in blood pressure

250. Which of the following is not a type of muscle tissue?

a. Skeletal
b. Smooth
c. Cardiac
d. Adipose

251. Which of the following organ systems has the purpose of producing movement through contraction?

a. Skeletal
b. Muscular
c. Cardiovascular
d. Respiratory

252. Which of the following terms means toward the front of the body?

a. Superior
b. Anterior
c. Inferior
d. Posterior

253. The brain is part of the:

a. Integumentary system
b. Nervous system
c. Endocrine system
d. Respiratory system

254. Which of the following is the name for the study of the structure and shape of the human body?

a. Physiology
b. Anatomy
c. Biology
d. Genetics

255. Which of the following is the name for the study of how parts of the body function?

a. Physiology
b. Anatomy
c. Biology
d. Genetics

256. Which of the below is the best definition for the term circulation?

a. The transport of oxygen and other nutrients to the tissues via the cardiovascular system
b. The force exerted by blood against a unit area of the blood vessel walls
c. The branching air passageways inside the lungs
d. The process of breathing in

257. Which of the following is not a type of connective tissue?

a. smooth
b. cartilage
c. adipose tissue
d. blood tissue

258. How many organ systems are there in the human body?

a. 4
b. 7
c. 11
d. 13

259. Which organ system includes the spleen?

a. Endocrine
b. Lymphatic
c. Respiratory
d. Digestive

260. Which of the following terms means close to the trunk of the body?

a. Superficial
b. Sagittal
c. Proximal
d. Distal

261. Which of the following does the integumentary system, the skin, NOT do?

a. Protect internal tissues from injury
b. Waterproofs the body
c. Helps regulate body temperature
d. Return fluid to the blood vessels

262. What does the term optic refer to?

a. The eye or vision
b. The ear or hearing
c. The mouth or tasting
d. The nose or smelling

263. What are groups of cells that perform the same function called?

a. tissues
b. plastids
c. organs
d. molecules

264. When does the nuclear division of somatic cells take place during cellular reproduction?

a. meiosis
b. cytokinesis
c. interphase
d. mitosis

265. Which group of major parts and organs make up the immune system?

a. lymphatic system, spleen, tonsils, thymus, and bone marrow
b. brain, spinal cord, and nerve cells
c. heart, veins, arteries, and capillaries
d. nose, trachea, bronchial tubes, lungs, alveolus, and diaphragm

266. What is the role of ribosomes?

a. make proteins
b. waste removal
c. transport
d. storage

267. Which of the following is an example of a tissue?

a. cortical bone
b. liver
c. mammal
d. hamstring

268. The adrenal glands are part of the

a. immune system
b. endocrine system
c. emphatic system
d. respiratory system

269. Hemoglobin transports oxygen from the lungs to the rest of the body, making oxygen available for cell use. What is hemoglobin?

a. an enzyme
b. a protein
c. a lipid
d. an acid

270. Which of the following statements describes the function of smooth muscle tissue?

a. It contracts to force air into and out of the lungs
b. It contracts to force air into and out of the stomach
c. It contracts to support the spinal column
d. It contracts to assist the stomach in the mechanical breakdown of food

271. Which of the following is not a product of respiration?

a. carbon dioxide
b. water
c. glucose
d. ATP

272. Of the following, the blood vessel containing the least-oxygenated blood is:

a. The aorta
b. The vena cava
c. The pulmonary artery
d. The capillaries

Answer Key and Explanations for Test #1

Reading Comprehension

1. C: The passage uses this word to discuss how your brain ignores the presence of your nose unless you specifically look at it. Thus, the best answer is choice C, *ignores*.

2. B: The retina is the part of the eye that processes the light that comes in through the lens and converts the visual signals into a form that the brain can more easily interpret. Thus, the best answer is choice B, *part of the eye*.

3. B: The final sentence reads, "Your brain works hard to make the world look continuous." This is another way of saying that visual perception is an active and *not a passive process*, making choice B the best answer.

4. A: If the reader follows the instructions given in the paragraph, the O and X in the middle of the passage can be used to demonstrate the blind spot in the visual field. Choice A is the best answer.

5. B: The passage spends most of its time explaining the way that visual perception works. Choice B is the best answer.

6. D: Much of the information in the passage is provided to show examples of how the brain fills in gaps in the visual field. Choice D is the best answer.

7. A: The author of the passage mentions the nose to demonstrate how the brain filters information out of the visual field. Choice A is the best answer.

8. B: The second paragraph states that the brain filters out information, which means that the brain does not perceive all activity in the visual field. In fact, it intentionally ignores some things in order to simplify the process of perception. Choice B is the best answer.

9. D: Of the given options, only choice D can be inferred from the passage. The passage states that parents should "try not to *feed into* oppositional behavior by reacting emotionally," which implies that reacting emotionally to defiant behavior can worsen it.

10. B: Choice B, "ODD is a complex condition" is the best answer out of the four that are given. It is the only choice that can be inferred from the passage as a whole.

11. A: Choice A is the best choice. *Oppositional* means uncooperative.

12. B: Choice B is the best interpretation of paragraph one. The passage states that many people exhibit ODD symptoms from time to time.

13. C: Choice C is the best choice. *Feed into* in this sentence means to encourage oppositional behavior.

14. C: Someone with a *low frustration tolerance* has a difficult time tolerating or dealing with frustration. Choice C is the best answer.

15. C: This passage is meant to inform the reader about ODD. Choice C is the best choice.

16. C: While some of these answer choices may contribute to ODD, the passage mentions only choice C, severe or unpredictable punishment.

17. A: The only statement directly supported by the passage is choice A.

18. B: As used in this passage, the word *parasite* means an organism that lives on or in another organism, which is choice B. Choice D is another definition for *parasite*, but does not fit the context of the word used in this passage.

19. C: According to the description of roundworms, they can live in the subcutaneous tissue of humans, which is choice C.

20. D: According to the first paragraph, protozoa are transmitted through food and water contaminated by fecal matter. It can then be inferred that clean sanitary conditions will prevent the spread of protozoa, which is choice D.

21. D: To answer this question, you will need to verify all three statements in the passage. All three of these statements are true and are supported by the passage.

22. D: Since the passage describes superstitions from days gone by about treating asthma, answer choice D is the correct one.

23. A: The reader can infer from the opening sentence that, if so many people have asthma today, many would probably have had asthma long ago as well. Even though the environment today is different than it was long ago, people would still have suffered from the condition. The sentence explains why people long ago may have needed to try homemade methods of treating the condition.

24. B: The purpose of the passage is to describe different measures that people took for asthma long ago, before the advent of modern medicine.

25. A: Of all the choices listed, only answer choice A is an example of misusing a drug. It is listed as one of the ways that drugs are misused in the middle of the passage. Taking more or less of a prescription drug than the amount that the doctor ordered can be harmful to one's health.

26. D: The passage does not say that ALL drugs add longevity. It says that drugs that are healthy and used properly add longevity. The word *all* makes the statement untrue.

27. C: The second paragraph of the passage notes that "up to one-third of people with peanut allergies have severe reactions." Since one-third is approximately 33%, choice C is correct.

28. D: The second paragraph of the passage notes that in 2008, Duke experts stated that they expect to offer treatment in five years. Five years from 2008 is 2013.

29. B: The last sentence in paragraph five lists the cuisines in which one should watch for peanuts. Italian is not listed.

30. A: The second sentence of the first paragraph states that peanut allergy is the most common cause of food-related death.

31. C: The passage implies that it is not always easy to know which foods have traces of peanuts in them and that it's important to make sure you know what you're eating. This is hard or impossible if you share someone else's food.

32. D: Paragraph two gives examples of symptoms of peanut allergies and, more specifically, examples of symptoms of anaphylaxis. A running or stuffy nose is given as a symptom of the former, but not of the latter.

33. B: All of the choices listed are names of diets given in the passage except choice B, Hunter Gatherer. Hunter-Gatherer refers to the prevailing methods of acquiring food at a prior time in human history, but it is not a name the passage gives for a diet.

34. B: Meat, vegetables, and nuts are all listed as foods on the Paleo diet, while dairy is listed as a food that is not allowed on the diet.

35. A: The passage notes that the idea behind the diet is that we are genetically adapted to the diet of our Paleolithic forebears.

36. B: The last sentence of the passage states that some studies support the idea of positive health benefits from the diet.

37. D: The directions indicate that the medication is *for relief of headaches*. The other choices are all contradicted within the passage.

38. C: The passage talks about what to do in case of stomach *upset*, so in this context, *upset* refers to a physical disorder.

39. C: The maximum number of pills one should take in a 24-hour period is 4. The directions instruct a person to contact a doctor after 24 hours.

40. B: The passage talks about the pain persisting, so in this context, *persists* most nearly means *continues*.

41. C: The 12 hours begins with the first pill that is taken. Four hours later, a second pill may be taken. After another four hours (eight hours after the first), a third pill may be taken. And finally, after another four hours (twelve hours in), a fourth may be taken. Thus, the answer is 4.

42. B: The second item on the list addresses this question. The tip recommends that those who drink whole milk gradually switch to fat-free milk. Since the question asks about ways to reduce saturated fat and calories, using skim milk in the place of water does not address the issue being raised.

43. A: The author uses a list format to organize the passage. There are no diagrams in the passage, and captions or labels would typically only be used with images or figures.

44. C: In the second item on the list, it states that reduced-fat milk is 2% milkfat, while low-fat milk is 1% milkfat, and skim milk is essentially fat free.

45. B: Statements I and II are both true statements about calcium rich foods. Canned fish, including salmon with bones, is recommended as a calcium rich food. Cheese is mentioned as a lactose-free alternative within the milk group. Statement III is false. According to the passage, condensed cream soups should be made with milk, not water.

46. D: The best choice for this question is choice D. The other options would clarify information for minor details within the passage and would provide little new information for the reader. However, food recommendations for those who do not consume milk products are listed under a separate heading, and lactose intolerance is the only reason listed. The reader can deduce that this is a main idea in the passage and the definition of "lactose intolerance" would help explain this main idea to the reader.

47. D: The author's style is to give facts and details in a bulleted list. Of the options given, you are most likely to find this style in a health textbook. A tourist guidebook would most likely make recommendations about where to eat, not what to eat. An encyclopedia would list and define individual foods. A friendly letter would have a greeting and a closing.

Vocabulary and General Knowledge

48. B: The best definition for the word *latent* is *dormant*. Something that is *latent* is unapparent but not necessarily nonexistent. For instance, a health condition can be latent without manifesting serious problems for many years. The word *thorough* suggests something that is complete and exhaustive, and this has no immediate connection to the word *latent*. The word *current* goes against the indication of the word *latent*, as the latter suggests something waiting for future events. The word *obvious* is an antonym of the word *latent*.

49. D: The meaning of the word *derelict* is *dilapidated*. A *derelict* building is one that is run-down, neglected, and *dilapidated*. The word *revived* is essentially an antonym to the word *derelict*, as it means resuscitated, rejuvenated, or brought back to life. Tentative means cautious or hesitant and redundant means superfluous or not needed to function.

50. C: The best definition for the word *aversion* is *abhorrence*. Some people have an *aversion* to country music; they *abhor* the sound of honky-tonk. *Attraction* is close to an antonym of *aversion*, since it means liking or being drawn to something. The meaning of *adequate* is acceptable or decent and the meaning of *antithesis* is opposite.

51. A: To *diffuse* is to *disseminate*, or spread around. The word *compress* suggests making something smaller and thus means the very opposite of *diffuse* and functions as an antonym. The word *distinct*, which means *unique* or *having qualities all its own*, has little similarity to the word *diffuse*. And while something might be *widened* to create a *diffusion*, the two words suggest related activities (or cause and effect) instead of similar meanings.

52. B: Something *anterior* is located near the *front*, so answer choice B offers the correct meaning of the word. Something *previous* comes before, but that does not necessarily mean the *front*. The word *crucial* has little relationship in meaning to the word *anterior*. The word *final* suggests the *end*, which is the very opposite of the *anterior*.

53. D: The word *rescinded* most nearly means *revoked*. The fisherman had his trout license *revoked*, so the permission he had to catch trout had been *rescinded*. *Acquired* and *restored* are close to antonyms of *rescinded* since they mean gaining or regaining something. *Denied* is close, but means refused or prohibited, not taken away.

54. A: In this case, the best definition for the word *comply* is *follow*. To *comply* is to go along with a request, or to *follow* orders or expectations. The word *affect* suggests a causal relationship, but this is not the same as a synonym. (For instance, to *comply* might be to *affect* something positively.) It might be possible to *depend* on someone or something to *comply*, but once again the relationship between the words is causal, so the words cannot have the same meaning. To *decline* is to refuse to *follow* a request/demand, so this is the opposite of *comply*.

55. A: The context of the sentence suggests that the CEO intends to show that he is still in charge, in spite of leadership problems. As a result, the word *maintain* offers the best synonym for *assert*. The words *prevent* and *censure* would indicate that the CEO is blocking his own authority, and this goes against the tone of the sentence. The word *accept* is positive regarding the CEO's authority, but it makes no sense for him to accept his own authority; that is for the employees to do (or not to do) after he has *asserted* it.

56. C: To *occlude* is to block, hinder, or *prevent*. The word *release* suggests the very opposite of *occlude* (as something that is released cannot be simultaneously blocked). The word *invade* also indicates an opposite within certain contexts. (For instance, a virus cannot *invade* cells if measures have been taken to *occlude* it.) The word *direct*, which indicates an order or command as a verb, has no clear relationship with the word *occlude*.

57. A: The sentence suggests that the colleague's remarks went beyond silly or unnecessary. If Eirinn feels that she should file a formal complaint, the colleague's remarks must have been *inappropriate*. If the comments were either *delicate* or *friendly*, Eirinn would almost certainly not be upset by them. The colleague might very well have delivered the *untoward* comments in an *eager* way, but eagerness alone is not unacceptable. The suggestion of offense is what leads Eirinn to pursue a formal complaint.

58. A: The best definition for the word *superficial* is *surface*. Something or someone that is *superficial* is focused only on appearances, or on what is on the *surface*. A wound that is *superficial* concerns only the *surface* of the skin. The word *backward* has little connection to the word *superficial*, even as an antonym. A *superficial* person, or even a *superficial* injury, might create problems that are *awkward*, but this is not the meaning of the word itself. Something that is *superficial* tends to be fairly empty in meaning or behavior and thus could not be described as *intense*.

59. D: The best definition for the word *inverted* is *reversed*. To *invert* is to turn inside out or show a different side, and the same could be said for something that is *reversed*. The word *credible* suggests believability, and this has no clear connection to *inversion*. The word *benign* means lacking in danger, and there is no immediate relationship between the meaning of *inversion* and the potential for danger. The word *forward* is directional, and this could be seen as an antonym for *inverted*: to *invert* is to present a different side, whereas something that is *forward* is likely showing its correct side(s).

60. A: The meaning of the word *void* is *emit*. *Voiding* is the process of releasing or removing the contents of something. *Emitting* is also releasing or sending out something. This is the closest meaning among the answer choices. To *determine* is to make a decision or make up one's mind about something. This has almost nothing to do with *voiding*. To *confirm* is to approve or agree. Again, there is no connection to the word *void* in this. The word *prevent* might be seen as a type of antonym in that *voiding* is releasing, while *preventing* is retaining. At the same time, the word *prevent* requires a context that is not essential with the word *void*, so these two words as well have little connection.

61. C: The context of the sentence suggests that Catriona is concerned about the danger of the fever, so it can be inferred that the word *adverse* means *negative*. Most people try to prevent fevers before they occur, and taking the child to the doctor once the fever has set in cannot be described as *preventive*. The word *auspicious* suggests something positive, and this contradicts the meaning inherent to the sentence. The word *reckless*, while negative in context, is not as closely related to *adverse* as the actual word *negative*. In fact, *reckless* suggests a deliberate attempt to do something dangerous, while the sentence suggests that Catriona is trying to prevent something dangerous.

62. A: The meaning of the word *contingent* is *dependent*. *Contingency* indicates a relationship between two (or more) items or events. For instance, going on vacation might be *contingent* upon not catching the flu. As this suggests *dependency*, answer choice A is correct. The connotation of the word *contingent* has little to do with *protection*, so answer choice B cannot be correct. The word *definite* suggests something that is absolute and unquestioned, whereas the word *contingent* suggests only possibility. The items or events that have inherent *contingencies* might very well be *intended*, but the word *intended* does not have the necessary suggestion of *dependency* to be correct.

63. B: Philippa is upset that her plans to leave the hospital early are foiled, so she wants the doctor to explain himself. In other words, she wants his *justification* for the decision. The word *description* indicates what the doctor will be doing (that is, *describing* his reasons), but this does not indicate fully that Philippa is looking more for a clear explanation of the doctor's *reasoning* rather than a mere *description*. The doctor might be *persistent* in his refusal to let Philippa leave the hospital early, but this is *why* she wants a *rationale* and does little to define the word *rationale*. It is *ambiguity* that Philippa does *not* want; the context suggests that she expects a clear explanation from the doctor.

64. D: The best definition for the word *patent* is *unconcealed*. Something that is *patent* is open, obvious, clear, and leaving no doubt. The word *inconspicuous*, suggesting something subtle or less obvious, means the very opposite of *patent*. The word *privileged* has no clear relationship to the word *patent*. Something that is *patent* might also be *carelessly* so, but this suggests a context that is not implied in the actual meaning of the word.

65. C: The best definition for the word *labile* is *fluctuating*. *Lability* indicates an ability to change quickly and rapidly, and the word *fluctuating* suggests constant movement or change. The word *external* is related to appearance or behavior, and while both of these might be *labile*, the underlying context of the word *external* has little relationship with the word *labile*. The word *meticulous* suggests the very opposite of the word *labile*. Something or someone *meticulous* is patient and takes the time to do something carefully and/or correctly. *Lability* indicates impatience more than *meticulousness*. The word *integral* indicates an inherent quality, and while *lability* might very well be *integral* to some things, the word *labile* means change, and the word *integral* does not.

66. B: The best definition for the word *impending* is *approaching*. An *impending* event is soon to arrive, and the word *approaching* indicates that something is on its way. The *impending* event might also be *demanding* on one's time or energy, but something *demanding* is not necessarily *impending*, so the relationship between the two words is too conditional. Something *impending* might also be *perilous*, and in literary terms it is often that *impending* events connote negative results. But the question asks for the *best* definition, and this is *approaching*. The word *producing* has little connection to the word *impending*, so answer choice D is incorrect.

67. A: The meaning of the word *cacophony* is *din*. The *cacophony* of the crowd of shoppers was eerily similar to the *din* of battle. *Dialogue* means conversation between two people, *divination* is fortune telling, and *diversity* means a variety.

68. B: The meaning of the word *boisterous* is *exuberant*. A *boisterous* individual is a lively person, full of energy and very animated. Some may find such people to be *obnoxious* as well, but that is not part of the definition of *boisterous*. *Masculine* means to have male characteristics and *robust* means sturdy or stable.

69. D: The context provided indicates that there was an awkward reception to the *comment*. The best definition for *acerbic* is *scathing*. The comment may have been *untruthful*, but that cannot be inferred from this sentence. If the comment were *solicitous*, it would have been kind and flattering, which is less likely to create an awkward social situation. It is also possible that the comment was *uncontrolled* if Bosworth has some form of Tourette's syndrome or something, but again, that is not a reasonable assumption from this context.

70. D: The best definition for the word *cloistered* is *sheltered*. When something is *cloistered* it is closed off from the surroundings or set apart in a protected place. *Sweetened* means that some form of sweetness has been added, *dampened* means that something has been made less intense or made a little wet, and *deafened* means that someone has their ability to hear reduced or inhibited in some way.

71. C: The best definition for the word *adsorb* is *accumulate*. To *adsorb* is to gather (such as particles) on the surface of something. Whereas *absorb* suggests a permeation, *adsorb* suggests an accumulation. The word *divide* indicates the very opposite of the word *adsorb*, since the process of *adsorption* gathers together. The word *process* has no immediate connection to the word *adsorb*. While *adsorption* is itself a *process*, *adsorbing* does not usually result in *processing* the particles that are gathered. Also, what is *adsorbed* might also be *contained*, but the suggestion of *containment* is conditional on other elements and not necessarily a part of the underlying meaning of the word *adsorb*.

72. B: The best definition for the word *compensatory* is *offsetting*. To *compensate* is to make up for something—in other words, to *offset* whatever is missing. Something *compensatory* might also be *corrupted*, but the presence of corruption has little to do with the meaning of the word *compensatory*. The word *varying* suggests change or fluidity, and this has no immediate connection to the word *compensatory*. The word *contradictory* indicates going against what is expected, and again this has no clear relationship with the meaning of *compensatory*.

73. A: The word *incompatible* suggests that two or more things cannot go together—that they are *conflicting*. The word *subsequent* suggests an event in which one thing follows another. The word *relevant* indicates that two things are related or appropriate for one another, so this could function as an antonym to *incompatible*. Similarly, the word *suitable* suggests that two things go together, so this is an antonym.

74. C: The word *lateral* indicates something that is sideways or *sideward*. There is no clear relationship between this and the word *positive*. The word *central* indicates a location other than the side, so it cannot be correct. The word *serious* suggests a quality about the word *lateral*, that a *lateral* injury can be *serious*, but this requires a qualification of the original word.

75. D: Something or someone described as *vivacious* would also be *vigorous* or full of life. *Viral* means related to viruses or spreading in a virus-like way. The word *vindictive* means acting with malicious and vengeful intent. The word *vitriolic* means bitter or caustic, often used to describe vicious criticism or malicious commentary.

76. C: The word *exiguous* suggests a lack or *inadequacy*. The word *superfluous* indicates an excessive amount, so this is an antonym for *exiguous*. The word *defective* indicates a failure, but this is not the same thing as a lack. A *defective* action can create an *exiguous* result, but this is a cause-and-effect relationship instead of a similarity in meaning. The word *eager* has no clear relationship with the word *exiguous*.

77. B: A claim that is *untenable* is *groundless* or without any support. The very opposite of an *untenable* claim would be a *logical* one, so answer choice A is an antonym. Something that is *opaque* is lacking in any transparency: there is no immediate relationship between *opaque* and *untenable*, except that an *untenable* claim could potentially be *opaque* as well. These are, however, entirely different qualities. Something *analogous* is similar or compatible, but there is nothing immediate in this to connect it with the word *untenable.*

78. D: To *placate* is to *comfort* or bring peace to someone or something. To *authorize* is to approve, so these words have no connection to each other in meaning. To *incite* is to create anger, so this is the very opposite of *placate.* To *clarify* is to make clear in explanation or meaning. As with *authorize*, there is nothing direct in the meaning to connect these words with each other.

79. A: To *inure* is to *toughen* someone or something against a current or future event. To *pretend* is to create an element of fantasy. While this is not a direct antonym to *inure*, there is a potential connection in opposites: something that is *inured* cannot *pretend* to ignore circumstances and must accept reality. To *anticipate* is to expect something to occur. One can *anticipate* an event by being *inured* to it, but this is a series of actions rather than a suggestion of a synonymous relationship. To *forget* is to lose track of something; a person who is *inured* cannot be allowed to *forget.*

80. C: The word *clement* indicates a situation (or individual) that is beneficent or *favorable.* In terms of opposites, *inclement* weather is bad weather that does not bode well for outdoor activities. Being *clement* means *not* being *difficult* or *angry*, so both answer choices are incorrect. A person who is *clement* can also be *righteous* in behavior, but the latter suggests a result of the former, indicating a cause-and-effect relationship instead of a relationship of synonyms.

81. A: To *malign* is to *harm* in a serious way. To *submit* is to give in and obey an order or expectation. There is no clear relationship between this and *malign*, so the words cannot be synonyms. To *improve* is to make better; to *malign* is to make worse, so the words are antonyms. To *conceive* is to create, so there is no direct relationship between this and *malign.*

82. B: To exist in *synergy* is to exist in a state of dwelling together comfortably or living in *harmony.* To *delay* is to prevent or slow down, and there is no immediate connection between this and *synergy.* A situation of *distress* indicates conflict, so this cannot be a state of *synergy.* A *hindrance* indicates a block, and this is the opposite of *synergy.*

83. D: To *recede* is to pull back or *retreat.* It can also suggest a diminishment, which would make the word *increase* an antonym. To *dilate* also indicates an increase or expansion, so this functions almost as an opposite. To *present* is to give or offer, and this has no clear connection with *recede.*

84. A: To *inflame* is to aggravate suddenly. For instance, banging an already sore knee could *inflame* the discomfort. As a result, the best definition is the word *worsen.* The word *ignite* has the hint of fire that is suggested by *inflame*, but in the latter case the word suggests a metaphorical condition or situation rather than anything connected literally to a flame. What is more, the word *ignite*, when metaphorical, indicates a cause (i.e., to *ignite* someone's interest), but it has no immediate connection to making something worse. To *lull* is the soothe or make better, so this is an antonym for *inflame.* To *inflame* something could be to *endanger* someone, but the relationship is causal rather than synonymous.

85. A: A *detriment* is a *drawback*, something negative that keeps a condition or situation from being as good as it should or could be. For instance, a cold could be a *detriment* for someone who hopes to enjoy a vacation. The word *retribution* suggests payback for some wrong that has been done, but there is no direct connection in this to a *drawback*—except that the *retribution* will almost certainly be a *drawback* for whoever is on the receiving end. The word *excitement* suggests eagerness or enthusiasm, and it is unlikely that a *detriment* could foster such an emotion. An *indulgence* is an excess of some kind (either of something tangible or of approval for behavior), and this suggests the very opposite of *detriment*—unless the *indulgence* ultimately represents a *detriment*, but that is causal and not indicated in the actual meaning.

86. C: The word *turgid* means swollen or *inflated*. This is not to be confused with *turbid*, which means *murky* (answer choice B). The word *intricate* suggests complexity, and there is nothing within the word *turgid* to indicate an immediate connection to this. The word *acceptable* means that something is good, and the word *turgid* reflects a condition that is unnatural or potentially serious, so answer choice D cannot be correct.

87. C: The word *paucity* indicates a *lack* or scarcity of something. The word *hunger* indicates a close possible meaning, in that hunger is the result of a *paucity* of food. But the word *result* in that statement indicates the real relationship, which requires a further explanation not immediate in the meaning. (In other words, *hunger* might result from *paucity*, but *paucity* does not always mean that the *lack* is one of food.) The word *affluence* suggests wealth or excess, so this functions as an antonym. The word *insistence* suggests an ongoing determination that something should be or occur, so there is no immediate connection in meaning to *paucity*.

88. D: To be *tractable* is to be *amenable*, that is open to suggestion and influence or able to be controlled. The word *interactive* means impacting one another or an exchange of information in two directions. To be *irresistible* is to be too desirable to be resisted. *Alluring* means attractive or inviting.

89. B: The word *austere* suggests meagerness or something/someone *stark* in choices, attitude, or behavior. The word *calm* is related to a condition of quietness, and while someone or something *austere* might also be *calm*, there is not enough in the meaning of each word to suggest a clear relationship. The word *dependable* indicates someone or something that can be relied upon. Again, there is not enough in the meaning to indicate a synonym with *austere*. The word *greedy* suggests a desire for excess, and this is the very opposite of the suggestion in *austere*.

90. D: To *delineate* is to *detail* something clearly. A mother who *delineates* instructions presents them so that her child knows exactly what to do. The very opposite of *delineate* would be *confuse*, since the goal of *delineating* is to avoid *confusion*. There is no clear connection in meaning with either *open* (as a verb) or *brag*.

91. B: Something *expedient* offers the best or most *practical* solution. The word *grateful* indicates a thankfulness for something, and there is nothing in this meaning to connect it with the meaning of *expedient*. Something *unprofitable* has no value, and this is the opposite of *expedient*, as the word *expedient* suggests a solution that is intended to offer immediate value. The word *substitute*, in suggesting an alternative, has a causal relationship with *expedient*: the *expedient* decision might also be the *substitute* option, but there is not enough in the meaning to make this direct connection.

92. B: To *facilitate* is to make something easier, or to *smooth* the way for something to occur. To *recast* is to start over; to *decide* is to make a choice. Neither of these has a direct relationship with the meaning of *facilitate*, so both are incorrect. To *thwart* is to hinder or make something difficult. This is opposite in meaning to *facilitate*.

93. C: The word *restive* describes someone who is *tense* about something and thus moving around (rather than resting comfortably). Someone who is *restive* might also be *frightened*, but he or she can also just be fidgety, so there is not enough suggestion of *fear* in *restive* to justify answer choice A. Someone who is *restive* might be so as the result of *hostility*, but this is a causal relationship instead of a synonymous one. Someone who is *apathetic* does not care about what is happening, and this indicates an opposite meaning of the word *restive*.

94. C: To have a *recourse* is to have another *option*. In other words, a *recourse* suggests a way out of a situation or an alternative choice. To *ambush* is to attack in surprise, so there is no real connection here to the meaning of *recourse*. An *obligation* is a required action, and a *recourse* is an alternative one, so these words suggest opposite meanings. A *proposal* is a presented idea, and while the *recourse* might come as the result of a *proposal* from someone, this is a cause-and-effect relationship.

95. A: To know the *impetus* for one's actions is to understand his or her *motivation(s)*, or reasons for doing something. A *diversion* is a distraction, so there is no clear relationship between this and the meaning of *impetus*. The word *authority* suggests a right of power, and again there is nothing in this to indicate the meaning of *impetus*. A *prevention* keeps one from doing something or keep something from occurring. There is nothing in this meaning to connect it to the meaning of *impetus*.

96. D: To know the *salient* points is to know what is *important*. The meaning of *salient* suggests information that is essential, and this goes beyond the meaning of *acceptable* (as allowable or adequate). Something *ordinary* is commonplace and does not indicate the degree of *importance* suggested in the meaning of *salient*. The word *peripheral* suggests the quality of being marginal or unimportant, so this is the opposite of *salient*.

97. C: Someone who is *laconic* tends to be *brief* in speech, getting right to the point and saying little else. Being *laconic*, or brief, is not the same as being *slow*, however, so the words do not have a close relationship in meaning. Being *laconic* also does not mean being *incomplete*: someone can be brief without leaving out important information. The word *tidy*, with its suggestion of cleanliness and organization, has no real connection to the meaning of *laconic*.

Grammar

98. A: The proper verb form to introduce volleyball is *playing*. Yoga is introduced with *doing* rather than *playing* because it is an activity rather than a game.

99. D: The word *every* is singular and requires a singular pronoun to represent it. In this case, *him* and *her* are both singular pronouns, but *him* is only objective case, while *her* may be objective or possessive. A possessive case pronoun is needed here, so the answer is *her*.

100. A: The phrasal verb "to put up with" means to have to deal with something or someone. None of the other phrases listed here form idiomatic expressions.

101. D: The simple future tense is [will + root form], in this case, *will study*. None of the other choices form a grammatically appropriate verb.

102. B: The part of speech needed in the blank is an adverb. Of the choices given, only *sympathetically* is an adverb. The other options are all adjectives.

103. A: The subject of this sentence is *a team*, which is a singular noun. Thus, the verb phrase for the sentence must also be singular in number. Of the choices given, only *is* meets that criterion.

104. B: In order to maintain consistency throughout the sentence, the verb phrase placed in the blank must be a simple past tense. Of the available options, only *showed up* qualifies.

105. B: The correct spelling is *presents*. All other words in the sentence are spelled correctly.

106. D: The correct spelling is *authority*. All other words in the sentence are spelled correctly.

107. B: The indefinite pronoun *each* is always singular, so a possessive pronoun representing it must also be singular. The only singular possessive pronoun among the available options is *her*.

108. A: The part of speech needed in the blank is an adverb. Of the choices given, only *tearfully* is an adverb. The other options are all adjectives.

109. B: The correct spelling is *misled*. All other answer options are either misspelled or would be grammatically incorrect in the sentence.

110. C: Since the action is taking place *tomorrow*, the correct choice must complete the future perfect form of the verb. Thus, *bring* is the correct word.

111. C: The word *each* is singular and requires a singular pronoun to represent it. By definition, a father is male, so *his* is the correct word to use.

112. B: To maintain a consistent verb tense throughout the sentence, the verb in the first half of the sentence must be a simple past tense. All the other answer options would make the verb tenses in the sentence inconsistent.

113. B: The part of speech needed in the blank is an adverb. Of the choices given, only *well* is an adverb. The other options are all adjectives.

114. C: The correct spelling is *niece*. All other words in the sentence are spelled correctly.

115. A: The correct spelling is *truly*. All other words in the sentence are spelled correctly.

116. B: The pronoun *Everyone* is singular and thus needs a singular verb. Among the verbs provided, only *needs* is both singular and makes sense in the context of the sentence. Stripped of the dependent clause, the sentence reads, "Everyone needs to see the new Manet exhibit." The verbs *should* and *must* both become unreadable with the addition of the infinitive phrase "to see" (while both would work if the "to" were removed), and the verb *have* is plural.

117. A: The possessive pronoun *Their* at the beginning of the sentence suggests third-person plurality, so answer choices B and D are immediately incorrect. (The first-person use of *we* and *I* excludes them as options.) The real choice comes down to *he and she* or *him and her*. In the sentence, the blank falls just after the start of a dependent clause, and this blank represents the subject of the dependent clause. As a result, the subjective case *he and she* must be correct.

118. B: After hearing about the party, Desmond knows that he *should have gone*. The expression *should have went* is never correct, under any circumstances. The expression *should go* makes little sense, as the context of the sentence indicates that the party has already occurred. The expression *should have been* also makes little sense, as the sentence indicates that Desmond wanted to *attend* the party, not *be* the party.

119. C: The word *who* is always used when referring to individual people, and the context of the sentence suggests that Loman is phoning a singular person *who* is the organizer. The word *that* is appropriate for groups, and the word *which* is appropriate for inanimate objects or things. The word *this* makes virtually no sense when added to the blank in the sentence.

120. D: Clearly, the cat belongs to the Millers, so it can be said to be *theirs* in the sentence. The context indicates that the cat is not Nessa's, so it is not *hers*. The Millers are clearly plural, so the cat is not *his*, singular. And as there is no first-person indication in the sentence, the cat cannot be *ours*.

No doubt, that is what the Millers would say, but because the sentence is third-person (and has no dialogue) the shift to first person is not appropriate here.

121. B: The presence of the conjunction *or* indicates the need for a singular verb. This sentence can be broken down with only one of the names to read correctly: "See to it that Derek collects..." or "See to it that Una collects..." The verb *are collecting* makes no sense when placed in the sentence. The plural verb *collect* does not work with the singular context implied by *or*. The verb *would collect* almost works but ultimately sounds strange when placed in the sentence.

122. A: The blank requires a second subject for the sentence, and the pronoun *she* is in the subjective case. The pronouns *him* and *me* are both in the objective case and thus do not fit the sentence correctly. It should be noted that the pronoun *they* is also subjective, but it is plural and thus does not fit the singular verb *knows*. While *Neither...nor...* is considered a singular expression, it can take a plural verb when the second subject is plural.

123. D: Because *was* is a being verb (those including *am, is, are, was, were*, etc.), it requires a subjective case pronoun to follow it. So, instead of "It was *him*," the expression is correctly "It was *he*." The possessive pronoun *his* makes no sense in the context of the sentence, and the reflexive *himself* could only follow the original pronoun. (For instance, "It was *he himself*." As this sounds fairly awkward, *himself* has no real place in this sentence.)

124. C: In this context, the word in the blank is the subject of the dependent clause and thus should be in the subjective case. Only *whoever* fits this requirement. To know for sure, simply substitute *whoever* with *he/she* and *whomever* with *him/her*. "He arrives first / she arrives first" makes far more sense than "him arrives first / her arrives first." So what about just using *who*? While technically in the subjective case, *who* sounds strange in the sentence, while *whoever* makes more sense. Why say, "The grand prize of $10,000 will be given to *who* arrives at the finish line first," when you can say, "The grand prize of $10,000 will be given to *whoever* arrives at the finish line first."

125. A: The blank in the sentence requires only a single preposition to create a prepositional phrase: "*off* the roof." Doubling up on prepositions (*off of, off from, away from*) is incorrect.

126. B: The word *committee* is a collective noun that can take either a singular or plural verb, depending on the context of the sentence. If there is agreement in the committee, the word is singular; if there is disagreement in the committee, the word is plural. For example, "The committee *agrees*..." but "The committee *disagree*..." In this question, the committee *were* in disagreement.

127. B: This question asks for the correct past tense usage of the verb *drink* when affixed to the helping verb *had*. The verb *drink* conjugates accordingly: *drink, drank, had drunk*. With the use of *had*, the correct choice is *drunk*. Fortunately, *had drunken* is never correct.

128. D: This question asks for the correct past tense usage of the verb *see* with the helping verb *has*. The verb *see* conjugates as such: *see, saw, had seen*. In this sentence, the use of *has* can take the place of *had* to indicate the correct usage: "What no eye has *seen*..."

129. C: The context of the sentence indicates that the ice-cream man has not yet arrived. The sentence projects into the future to say that *when* he arrives the children *will be excited*. In the latter case, the verb also suggests a future context and is thus correct. The past tense *were excited* makes no sense in the sentence. The conditional tenses *would be excited* and *would have been excited* also make little sense in the context of future activities that are presented as definite.

130. A: This sentence requires a slightly unexpected combination of future and continuous past tenses. The speaker points out that when something happens in the future (i.e., the completion of the final pose), something will then have been in the process of occurring for two hours. In this case, the verb *will have been doing* successfully indicates both cases to make the sentence read correctly. The fully future *will do* and *will be doing* do not work without some hint of a continuous past sentence as well. The verb *would be doing* is conditional, but the rest of the context of the sentence does not have enough suggestion of conditional activity to make this verb work. The speaker is confident of completing the yoga routine; the verb needs to indicate this. (The use of *If* at the beginning of the sentence instead of *Once* would provide the sense of the conditional.)

131. A: The blank space requires the start of a dependent clause. In this case, the word *that* is most correct. The word *which* is more correct to introduce a clause that is not necessarily essential to the sentence. Because the sentence makes little sense without the clause, the word *that* is necessary to introduce it. The word *than* suggests comparison, so it has no place introducing a dependent clause. The word *who* should introduce a phrase or clause that refers to a person, and since the sentence refers to the inanimate *vacation plan*, the word *who* is not correct.

132. D: The sentence requires two adverbs: *really badly*. The adverb *badly* modifies the verb *performed*, while the adverb *really* modifies the adverb *badly* to answer the question *How?* All other answer choices are either entirely correct or only partially correct. The words *real* and *bad* are adjectives without the addition of *-ly*, so both cannot be correct to modify a verb and an adverb.

133. D: No preposition is necessary at the end of the question. The directional word *Where* indicates location, so the addition of *to*, *from*, or *at* is unnecessary and makes the sentence grammatically incorrect. What is more, the use of *from* and *at* makes little sense in the context of the question.

134. C: The verb *have* is correct here to complete the verb: *should have*. The entire expression is a verb, so the preposition *of* cannot be correct to complete it. The verb *be* makes no sense in the context of the sentence. The verb *has* does not fit the use of *I* or the addition of *should*. (The verb *should* always requires the form *have*; the form *has* is never correct with it.)

135. A: The comma belongs after the dependent clause, so it is correct between the words *mother* and *he*: *When Finn called his mother, he did not tell her about all of his plans*. The comma between *called* and *his* makes little sense, as there is no need for a pause between these words. In the same way, the comma between *not* and *tell* breaks the sentence up awkwardly, so it cannot be correct. The comma after the word *When* is incorrect because the comma belongs after the entire dependent clause instead of just after the relative adverb.

136. D: The context of the sentence indicates that Professor Howard is grading the papers of all thirty-five students, so the sentence requires the possessive of a plural word. The correct form would be *students'*. The form *student's* would suggest the possessive of a singular word. The word *students* is simply plural but not possessive, and the sentence indicates the possession of *papers* belonging to *students*. The form *student's* is never correct.

137. D: The sentence requires an adverb form to modify the verb *did*, and the only correct adverb form among the answer choices is *well*. The words *good* and *great* are adjectives. The word *worse* makes little sense as it contradicts the context of the sentence: most teachers do not praise their students for doing *worse* on something.

138. C: The comma belongs before the coordinating conjunction to indicate the combination of two independent clauses. In this case, the coordinating conjunction is *but*, so the correct version is: *Olaf* *planned to see the movie, but he could not go after he caught the flu*. The comma after the coordinating conjunction is never correct if there is no comma before the coordinating conjunction. (A comma after the coordinating conjunction is correct—when there is also one before it—if there is a required pause at the start of the new independent clause.) The comma between *movie* and *he* removes the conjunction *but* and thus functions as a comma splice, incorrectly joining two independent clauses. The semicolon between *but* and *he* makes no sense in its placement.

139. A: The single apostrophe is appropriate because the context of the sentence suggests that Melissa and Caroline share the dorm room. If they were in separate rooms, then the form *Melissa's and Caroline's* would be acceptable, but the sentence indicates that Maura only knocks on the door of one room. The form *Melissa's and Caroline* reads awkwardly by assigning the possession to the first person and leaving the reader unsure of what this means. The lack of apostrophes altogether also makes little sense by placing the two names in the middle of the sentence but not indicating clearly their relationship to the dorm room.

140. C: The form *1980s* is correct without the apostrophe, since it is plural instead of possessive. Any form with the apostrophe at the end (*1980's* and *1980s'*) is incorrect to indicate a plural form. The form with the apostrophe at the beginning of the expression (*'1980s*) would only be correct if the *19* were dropped at the beginning (*'80s*), because the apostrophe here suggests that something has been removed from the expression—much like a contraction.

141. C: The context of the sentence indicates contrast: Jean intended to hold the picnic, *but* the rain prevented it from happening. The conjunction *and* suggests addition that makes the sentence sound more confusing. The word *however* is not a conjunction and creates a run-on sentence when added just after a comma (and without a coordinating conjunction). The word *or* suggests the presence of options or alternatives, and this makes little sense in the context of the sentence.

142. B: If the instructor intends to prevent cheating, the study notes will have to be collected *before* the exam. Collecting them *during* or *after* the exam would only increase the potential for the students to consult them. (And the context of the sentence suggests that consulting the study notes would qualify as cheating.) Collecting the study notes *upon* the exam makes almost no sense. It would be possible to collect them *upon the start* of the exam, but as the sentence does not include the expression *the start*, the preposition *upon* does not work here.

143 C: This is a rare case when both forms of *effect* (verb and noun) are used correctly in the sentence. The word *effect* is used as a verb when it expresses a specific desire to cause something to occur: *effect* a compromise, *effect* a change. The noun form of *effect* is the result of the change, so both forms are correct in this sentence. The form *affect* is incorrect in both places in the sentence.

144. A: The context of the sentence suggests that Eleanora cannot *accept* (or receive) gifts, *except* (or only) from colleagues and only when the gift is a birthday gift. This requires that *accept* go in the first blank and *except* go in the second blank.

145. D: The form *ensure* indicates a desire to guarantee that something occurs. The form *insure* is related only to insurance. In other words, a homeowner will *insure* a home against fire to *ensure* that he or she is covered if a fire breaks out. Answer choice D places the forms in the correct order for the sentence: *ensure, insure*.

146. B: Since the second part of this sentence goes on to list examples that help support the point made in the first sentence, "for instance" is the best transitional phrase.

147. C: The second part of the sentence adds additional evidence to prove the claim made in the first part. "In fact" is the best transition to introduce supporting evidence.

Mathematics

148. A: The word "percent" literally means per hundred; a percentage is a fraction over 100. 25% is therefore equal to $\frac{25}{100}$. To find a percentage of a number, you can multiply the number by the percentage and then divide by 100. 25% of 400 is therefore $400 \times 25 \div 100 = 100$.

Alternatively, you can remember that 25% is equal to one quarter—this is one of a few percentages that is simple enough to be worth committing to memory. Thus 25% of 400 is one quarter of 400; $400 \div 4 = 100$.

149. C: The **reciprocal** of a number is the number which, when multiplied by the first number, makes a product of 1. In other words, it's one divided by the first number. (Zero has no reciprocal.) For a fraction, you can find the reciprocal easily by just switching the numerator and denominator—turning the fraction "upside-down". For instance, the reciprocal of $\frac{2}{3}$ is $\frac{3}{2}$: $\frac{2}{3} \times \frac{3}{2} = 1$. An integer can be written as a fraction with a denominator of 1: $6 = \frac{6}{1}$. Therefore, we can find the reciprocal of 6 by swapping the numerator and denominator of $\frac{6}{1}$ to get $\frac{1}{6}$.

150. B: The average rate of change of a quantity over a period of time is equal to the change in the quantity divided by the time. In this case, the change in temperature is $145\ °\text{F} - 32\ °\text{F} = 113\ °\text{F}$. This occurs over four hours, so the average rate of change is $113\ ° \div 4\ \text{hr} = 28.25\ °\text{F/hr}$.

151. A: We can find the cost of the pens and staplers separately and then add the two together. We are purchasing 240 pens, and they cost $2.35 per pack. Since there are six pens per pack, we can find the number of packs needed by dividing the number of pens by six: 240/6 = 40. (If we had come up with a fraction, we would have rounded up, since we presumably can't purchase a partial pack, but in this case 240 is evenly divisible by 6 anyway.) So the cost of the pens is equal to 40 packs × \$2.35/pack = \$94. Similarly, we need 6/2 = 3 sets of staplers, which will cost 3 sets × \$12.95/set = \$38.85. \$94 + \$38.85 = \$132.85.

152. D: A percentage is equal to a fraction over 100: $p\% = \frac{p}{100}$. That means to find a number x that corresponds to $p\%$, we need to solve $x = \frac{p}{100}$, which just comes out to $p = 100x$. In other words, to convert a decimal to a percentage, we just multiply by 100. So to find the percentage that corresponds to 0.45, we just multiply $0.45 \times 100 = 45$: 0.45 = 45%. (Note that $45\% = \frac{45}{100} = 0.45$, as desired.)

153. B: If the vitamin lost a certain quantity of calcium, it means the amount of calcium was reduced by that amount. So we can subtract that amount from the original amount of calcium to find the amount that remains. 500 mg – 325 mg = 175 mg.

154. C: Each dose contains 4 mg, and you have to give the patient a total of 20 mg. So we can find out how many doses you need to give the patient by finding out how many times 4 mg goes into 20 mg: 20 mg ÷ 4 mg = 5. So the patient needs 5 doses. Now, to find the total volume of the doses, you can multiply the volume of each dose by the number of doses. Each dose has a volume of 5 mL, so the total volume is 5 mL × 5 = 25 mL.

155. A: In a decimal number, the digit just before the decimal point represents the unit space, or the ones space. (For a number without a decimal, the last digit is in the ones space.) Each space to the left represents a larger space by a factor of ten: so the digit left of the ones place is the tens place, the digit left of that is the hundreds space, and so on. Each space right represents a *smaller* space by a factor of ten: so the digit to the right of the ones place (the digit just right of the decimal point) is the tenths place, the digit to the right of that is the hundredths space, and so on.

In this case, we're asked for the tenths place, which as we've just seen is the digit just right of the decimal point: 2. The 3 represents the ones space, the 4 represents the tens space, and the 5 represents the hundredths space.

156. C: A percentage represents a number of hundredths, so to convert a decimal to a percentage, we multiply by 100. (This is equivalent to moving the decimal point two spaces to the right, adding zeroes as necessary.) In this case, then, the percentage we need is $1.25 \times 100 = 125$; 1.25 is equal to 125%. That's greater than 100%, but that makes sense, because $100\% = 1$ and 1.25 is greater than one.

157. B: The fraction is simply equal to the part over the whole. In this case, if the average person drinks eight 8-oz glasses of water during a day, then the total amount of water the person drinks is 8×8 oz $= 64$ oz. If we now want to know what fraction 12.8 oz is of this number, we write 12.8 oz / 64 oz, or just $\frac{12.8}{64}$.

This, however, is a messy fraction; we'd like to simplify and get rid of the decimals. We can rewrite a fraction in equivalent form by multiplying or dividing both the numerator and denominator by the same number. Multiplying by 10 gets rid of the decimal, leaving $\frac{128}{640}$. Now, both the numerator and denominator are even, so we can divide them both by 2, leaving $\frac{128 \div 2}{640 \div 2} = \frac{64}{320}$. They're still even, so we can repeat the process, and keep repeating until they no longer have a common factor, yielding $\frac{32}{160}$, then $\frac{16}{80}$, then $\frac{8}{40}$, then $\frac{4}{20}$, then $\frac{2}{10}$, and finally $\frac{1}{5}$. (We could have done this in fewer steps by dividing by larger factors, but those larger common factors are less obvious.)

For this problem, though, there's a significant shortcut: all of the answer choices have a 1 in the numerator, which we know we can get by dividing the numerator by itself. So we can just divide the numerator and denominator by 12.8: $\frac{12.8 \div 12.8}{64 \div 12.8} = \frac{1}{5}$.

158. D: A percentage is a number of hundredths, thus $33\% = \frac{33}{100}$. So to find a given percentage of a number, we can just multiply the number by the corresponding fraction: 33% of 300 = $\frac{33}{100} \times 300 = \frac{9900}{100} = 99$.

159. D: To find the amount of water you need to add, you can subtract the amount you've already added from the total required. In this case, that means $\frac{4}{5} - \frac{1}{3}$. To add or subtract fractions, it's necessary to rewrite them so that their denominators match; we then subtract the numerators, keeping the same denominator. We can rewrite a fraction in an equivalent form by multiplying the numerator and denominator of the fraction by the same number.

For us to subtract the fractions, their new denominator should be the lowest common multiple of the original denominators: that is, the smallest number that is divisible by the denominators of both fractions. In this case, the lowest common multiple of 3 and 5 is 15. We therefore rewrite $\frac{4}{5}$ as $\frac{4\times3}{5\times3}=\frac{12}{15}$, and $\frac{1}{3}$ as $\frac{1\times5}{3\times5}=\frac{5}{15}$. The difference is then $\frac{12}{15}-\frac{5}{15}=\frac{7}{15}$.

160. A: To add or subtract fractions, we have to rewrite them so that they have the same denominator. We then subtract the numerators, keeping the same denominator (and simplifying if possible). This new denominator is the lowest common multiple of the original fractions: the smallest number that is divisible by both the original denominators. The lowest common multiple of 2 and 4 is 4, so we need to rewrite both fractions with this denominator. $\frac{3}{4}$ already has the correct denominator; to rewrite $\frac{1}{2}$ we multiply both sides of the fraction by 2: $\frac{1}{2}=\frac{1\times2}{2\times2}=\frac{2}{4}$. Our subtraction problem then becomes $\frac{3}{4}-\frac{2}{4}=\frac{1}{4}$.

161. B: The total number of students in the class is 48, and 32 are female, which means the number of male students is $48-32=16$. The fraction of students that are male is therefore $\frac{16}{48}$.

There are two ways to proceed from here. We can convert the fraction into a decimal by dividing, using a calculator if necessary: $16\div48=0.3333\ldots$; multiplying by 100 gives approximately 33.

In this case, however, there's another way to solve the problem. We can reduce the fraction by dividing both sides of the fraction by 16: $\frac{16}{48}=\frac{16\div16}{48\div16}=\frac{1}{3}$. This is a common enough fraction that the equivalent percentage may be worth committing to memory: $\frac{1}{3}$ is approximately equal to 33%.

162. B: The necessary formula is given in this problem, so all we have to do is put the given numbers into the given formula. It is, however, important to note that the formula requires the child's age in months, whereas the given age is in years. That's easy to convert, however: $2\text{ years}\times12\text{ months/year}=24\text{ months}$. Putting this into the formula, we get $\frac{24\times15\text{ mg}}{150}=\frac{360\text{ mg}}{150}=2.4\text{ mg}$.

163. C: One way to subtract mixed numbers is to subtract the integer and fractional parts separately. To subtract the fractions, we first have to convert both fractions to the lowest common denominator: in this case, 8. So we can rewrite $\frac{1}{2}$ as $\frac{1\times4}{2\times4}=\frac{4}{8}$. Subtracting the fractional parts yields $\frac{4}{8}-\frac{3}{8}=\frac{1}{8}$. (If the right fraction had been larger, we would have had to borrow one from the left integer, but in this case that isn't necessary.) Subtracting the integer parts gives $7-5=2$. So the solution to the problem is $2\frac{1}{8}$.

Alternatively, we can first convert the mixed numbers to improper fractions: $7\frac{1}{2}=\frac{7\times2+1}{2}=\frac{15}{2}$, and $5\frac{3}{8}=\frac{5\times8+3}{8}=\frac{43}{8}$. As above, we rewrite the fractions with the same denominator: $\frac{15}{2}=\frac{15\times4}{2\times4}=\frac{60}{8}$. Now, $\frac{60}{8}-\frac{43}{8}=\frac{17}{8}$. Finally, we convert this improper fraction back into a mixed number: 8 goes into 17 2 times with a remainder of 1, so $\frac{17}{8}=2\frac{1}{8}$.

164. A: Recall that a percentage is a number of hundredths, thus $20\%=\frac{20}{100}=0.2$. To find 20% of a number, we multiply the number by 0.2. In that case, therefore, we're looking for the number that, when multiplied by 0.2, yields 35. That would be $35\div0.2=175$.

165. D: We could multiply this out with a calculator, but there is an even simpler way to solve this problem. Note that one of the numbers in the product is zero. Zero multiplied by anything is zero; no matter how many other numbers are multiplied together, if one of the factors is zero, the product is zero. Therefore, we know immediately that the product of this series of numbers is zero without having to use a calculator or do any lengthy calculations.

166. B: We could easily solve this problem with a calculator, but it's also possible to solve it without one. We could solve it as a regular long division problem, but we have to first get rid of the decimal point in the divisor. We can do that by moving the decimal point the same number of spaces in both the divisor and the dividend. Moving the decimal point one space to the right gives $79.5 \div 15$. Now, we can proceed with a regular long division, putting the decimal point in the quotient directly above the decimal point in the dividend:

$$\begin{array}{r} 5.3 \\ 15\overline{)79.5} \\ \underline{75} \\ 4\,5 \\ \underline{4\,5} \\ 0 \end{array}$$

167. C: To convert a fraction to a decimal, just divide the numerator by the denominator: $\frac{7}{10} = 7 \div 10 = 0.7$ (as can be verified either by using a calculator or by performing the division by hand). Alternatively, we can remember that the first digit after the decimal point is the tenths place, so any proper fraction with a 10 in the denominator is just the digit in the numerator after a decimal point: $\frac{1}{10}$ is 0.1, $\frac{3}{10}$ is 0.3, etc., and so $\frac{7}{10}$ is 0.7.

168. C: To convert a fraction to a decimal, just divide the numerator by the denominator: $\frac{4}{8} = 4 \div 8 = 0.5$ (as can be verified either by using a calculator or by performing the division by hand). Alternatively, we can observe that the fraction $\frac{4}{8}$ can be reduced, since both the numerator and denominator are divisible by 4: $\frac{4}{8} = \frac{4 \div 4}{8 \div 4} = \frac{1}{2}$, and $\frac{1}{2}$ is a common enough fraction that it's worth remembering its decimal and percentage equivalents: $\frac{1}{2} = 50\% = 0.5$.

169. A: When adding a positive and negative number, the absolute value of the result is equal to the *difference* of the absolute values of the individual numbers: $32 - 7 = 25$. The sign of the result is the same as the sign of the number with the *larger* absolute value. In this case, $|32| > |7|$, so since the 32 is negative so is the result: –25.

We can also visualize this with a number line. Negative numbers are to the left of zero on the number line; positive numbers are to the right. Adding a positive number moves us right on the number line; adding a negative number moves us left. We start at –32, to the left of zero, and move seven places to the right, bringing us closer to zero, and specifically to –25.

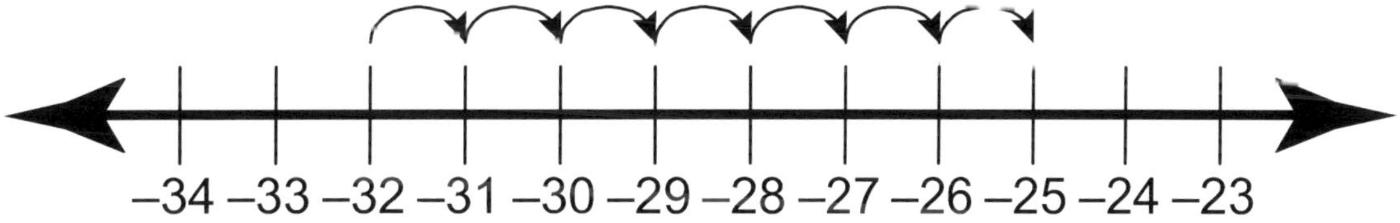

170. B: A percentage is equal to a number of hundredths: thus 41% is equal to $\frac{41}{100}$. To convert a percentage to a decimal, therefore, you just have to divide the percentage by 100—which is equivalent to moving the decimal point two places to the left. (If the number has no decimal point, you can consider the decimal point to be just to the right of the final digit.) In this case, $\frac{41}{100} = 0.41$.

171. B: This is a simple addition problem. Start with the ones column (on the right). Add the figures 8+1, 4+1, 2+3 to get the answer 559.

172. C: This is a simple addition problem with carrying. Start with the ones column and add 0+1. Write down the 1 and add the digits in the tens column: 8+3. Write down the 1 and add the 1 to the digits in the hundreds column. Add 9+1+1 and write down 1. Add the 1 to the digits in the thousands column. Add 3+7+1 and write down the 1. Add the 1 to the digits in the ten-thousands column. Add 1+1 and write down 2 to get the answer 21,011.

173. B: This is a simple subtraction problem. Start with the ones column and subtract 7-6, then 3-1, then 5-3, then 8-6 to get 2,221.

174. C: This is a multiplication problem with carrying. Start with the ones column. Multiply 2 by each digit above it beginning with the ones column. Write down each product: going across-- it will read 1268. Now multiply 7 by each of the digits above it. Write down each product: going across, the figure will read 4501. Ensure that the 1 is in the tens column and the other numbers fall evenly to the right. Now add the numbers like a regular addition problem to get 46,296.

175. D: This is a simple division problem. Divide 63 into 181. It goes in 2 times. Write 2 above the 1 and subtract 136 from 181. The result is 55. Bring down the 4. Divide 63 in 554. It goes in 8 times. Write 8 above the first 4 and subtract 504 from 554 to get 50. Bring down the 4. Divide 63 into 504. It goes in 8 times.

176. C: This is a simple addition problem. Line up the decimals so that they are all in the same place in the equation, and see that there is a 3 by itself in the hundredths column. Then add the tenths column: 6+3+5 to get 14. Write down the 4 and carry the 1. Add the ones column: 3 plus the carried 1. Write down 4. Then write down the 1.

177. D: This is multiplication with decimals. Multiply 3 by 9 to get 27. Put down the 7 and carry the 2. Multiply 3 by 1 to get 3. Add the 2. Write 5 to the left of 5. Multiply the 2 by the 9 to get 18. Enter the 8 and carry 1. Multiply 2 by 1 to get 2. Add 1 and write down 3. Add the two lines together, making sure that the 8 in the bottom figure is even with the 5. Get 437. Count 4 decimal points over (2 from the top multiplier and 2 from the second multiplier) and add a 0 before adding the decimal.

178. C: To solve, divide 0.08 into 0.3. Move the decimal in 0.08 over 2 places to make it an 8. Because this decimal point was moved 2 places, it must be done to the other decimal too. 0.3 becomes 30.0. Now divide 8 into 30. Put a 3 above 0 (ensure that the decimal is beside it) and subtract 24 from 30. Bring down the 0 and put it beside the 6. Divide 8 into 60. Put 7 above the 0 and subtract 56 from 60. Bring down the 0 and put it beside the 4. Divide 8 into 40. Put 5 beside the 7.

179. C: Count from the 5: tenths, hundredths, thousandths.

180. A: This is a simple subtraction problem involving decimals. Line up the decimals and subtract 7 from 3. Since 7 is a larger number than 3, borrow ten from the 4. Cross out the 4 and make it 3. Now subtract 7 from 13 to get 6. Subtract 1 from 3 and get 2. Place the decimal point before the 2.

181. D: Circle the 4 in the hundredths place. Look at the digit in the thousandths place. Since that digit is more than 5, the 4 is rounded up becoming a 5.

182. A: To add fractions, ensure that the denominator (the number on the bottom) is always the same common denominator. Since there is not common denominator in this case, change both fractions to 14ths. 1/2 equals 7/14. 1/7 equals 2/14. Now add the whole numbers: 2+3 = 5 and the resulting fraction become 9/14.

183. B: To subtract fractions, ensure that the denominator (the number on the bottom) is the same. Having the same "common denominator" is essential to solving the problem. Since there is no common denominator in this case, t, change both fractions to 36ths. 1/9 equals 4/36. 1/4 equals 9/36. The equation now looks like this: $3\frac{4}{36} - 1\frac{9}{36}$. Change the 3 to 2 and add 36 to the numerator (the top number) so that the fractions can be subtracted. The equation now looks like this: $2\frac{40}{36} - 1\frac{9}{36}$. Subtract: $1\frac{31}{36}$

184. A: To multiply mixed numbers, you must first create improper fractions. Multiply the whole number by the denominator, and then add the numerator.

$$3\frac{1}{8} = \frac{25}{8}$$

The problem will look like this: $\frac{28}{5} \times \frac{19}{3} \times \frac{12}{5} = \frac{5700}{120} = 47\frac{1}{2}$

185. A: To divide fractions, change the second fraction to its reciprocal (its inverse) and multiply: $\frac{1}{8} \times \frac{5}{4}$

186. B: The denominator has been multiplied by 4 to get 20. Think of what number multiplied by 4 totals 12.

187. C: Divide the numerator and denominator by 17.

188. A: Since all the answers have a 7 as the whole number, multiply 7 x 14. The answer is 98. The remainder is 1.

189. D: Divide 3 by 50 to get 0.06 or 6%.

190. C: Divide 60 by 5 to get 12. Multiply 12 by 3.

191. A: Rewrite the problem as 40 × 0.5% and solve. Since the answer choices are not in percent form, do not forget to divide by 100 to convert from percentage to decimal.

192. D: Divide 2 by 10 (not 10 by 2). Multiply by 100 to get answer in % form.

193. C: To change a fraction to a percent, multiply it by 100:

$$\frac{3}{5} \times 100\% = 60\%$$

194. A: To solve, first write the fraction as $\frac{15}{100}$. Reduce by dividing numerator and denominator both by 5.

195. B: To solve change 1.25% to a decimal: 0.0125. Now add an x for the question mark: $0.0125x = 1.5$. Divide 1.5 by 0.0125.

196. C: To solve, rewrite the equation with a decimal in place of the percent:

$$8 = 0.25x$$

$$x = \frac{8}{0.25} = \frac{800}{25} = 32$$

197. C: To solve, change the percent to a decimal:

$$0.40x = 18$$

$$x = \frac{18}{0.40} = \frac{180}{4} = 45$$

Biology

198. A: All organisms begin life as a single cell.

199. B: The process by which organisms use energy is called metabolism.

200. D: Only cells with a membrane around the nucleus are called eukaryotes.

201. C: The two types of cellular transport are active (which requires the cell to invest energy) and passive (which does not require the cell to expend energy).

202. A: Aerobic means in the presence of oxygen.

203. B: When both parents give offspring the same allele, the offspring is homozygous for that particular trait.

204. C: Genetics is the study of heredity.

205. B: Scientists suggest that evolution has occurred through a process called natural selection.

206. D: The cellular hierarchy starts with the cell, the simplest structure, and progresses to organisms, the most complex structures.

207. B: A hypertonic solution is a solution with a higher particle concentration than in the cell, and consequently lower water content than in the cell. Water moves from the cell to the solution, causing the cell to experience water loss and shrink.

208. C: Interphase is the period when the DNA is replicated (or when the chromosomes are replicated) and is the longest part of the cell cycle.

209. B: Recessive alleles are represented by lower case letters, while dominant alleles are represented by upper case letters,

210. C: Dominant genes are always expressed when both alleles are dominant (BB) or when one is dominant and one is recessive (Bg). In this case, ¾ or 75% will have brown eyes.

211. A: The trait Ll describes the genotype of the person or the traits for the genes they carry. It is heterozygous because it contains a dominant gene and a recessive gene. Tallness is the phenotype of the person or the physical expression of the genes they carry, because L for tallness is the dominant gene.

212. C: Arthritis is a type of non-communicable disease because it is not passed from person to person.

213. D: All living organisms on Earth utilize the same triplet genetic code, in which a three-nucleotide sequence called a codon provides information corresponding to a particular amino acid to be added to a protein. In contrast, many organisms, especially certain types of bacteria, do not use oxygen. These organisms live in oxygen-poor environments, and may produce energy through fermentation. Other organisms may live in dark environments, such as in caves or deep underground. Many organisms reproduce asexually by budding or self-fertilization, and only the most evolutionarily-advanced organisms make use of neurotransmitters in their nervous systems.

214. B: The nitrogenous bases found in DNA are thymine, guanine, adenine, and cytosine. Uracil is the base used in mRNA in the place of thymine.

215. A: Water is a polar substance and so does not interact well with nonpolar compounds (think: oils). Enzymes are actually an example of tertiary proteins not secondary. Exergonic reactions create energy, rather than use it up.

216. C: Ribosomes are small intracellular organelles that build proteins. The proteins are then sent to the Golgi apparatus for modification and packaging into their final form. The endoplasmic reticulum is responsible for transporting proteins through the cell. Lysosomes are small pouches in the cytoplasm that contain digestive enzymes. These vacuoles help the cell break down old or worn out organelles or cellular material.

217. C: Prokaryotes are single-celled organisms, which do not have nuclei. Their genetic material is condensed in the cytoplasm of the cell. Prokaryotes do have ribosomes and a cell membrane. Most also have a cell wall that aids in protection of the organism.

218. A: During metaphase, the chromosomes begin to line up in the center of the cell as the spindle fibers attach themselves to the centromeres on one end and the centrioles on the other. Next, anaphase occurs as the chromosomes are split into two identical sister chromatids. Prophase is the first stage of mitosis and refers to when the cell prepares for division: the nuclear membrane begins to break down, centrioles start migrating to the end of the cell, and the DNA becomes organized and prepared for mitosis. Telophase is the last stage of mitosis and occurs when the two chromatids start separating and the new nuclear envelopes begin to reform around the new nuclei.

219. B: There are four stages of Interphase:

a. G_1 (the stage immediately after the new daughter cells have been formed – the resting phase)
b. S (the stage of rapid DNA synthesis and replication),
c. G_2 (the stage of rapid cellular growth in preparation for mitosis), and
d. M (mitosis).

220. D: Meiosis is the process where one diploid (2n) cell will eventually divide to form four haploid (n) cells, which have half the number of chromosomes as the body cells. These haploid cells are gametes, not body cells.

221. D: The Krebs cycle actually occurs twice per molecule of glucose, as glucose is broken into two molecules of pyruvate, which are each eventually turned into acetyl-coA before entering the Krebs cycle. This cycle is an aerobic process, and it takes place in the inner part of the mitochondria.

222. C: The bulk of the energy released from ATP occurs when the first phosphate molecule breaks off AT to form ADP and phosphate. This is a hydrolysis reaction, meaning that it is facilitated by the water to break the bonds between phosphate and ADP. ATP is re-formed using a dehydration reaction, where water is removed from ADP and phosphate and they form a chemical bond.

Chemistry

223. B: Mass is not the same as weight; rather, mass is the quantity of matter an object has.

224. C: There are three common states of matter: gases, liquids, and solids. The fourth state of matter, not commonly encountered on earth, is plasma.

225. D: An element is a substance that cannot be broken into simpler types of matter.

226. D: The two types of measurement important in science are quantitative (when a numerical result is used) and qualitative (when descriptions or qualities are reported).

227. D: A solid turns to a liquid by melting, and a liquid turns to a gas by vaporization.

228. B: An atom with an electrical charge is called an ion.

229. C: When atoms from two elements combine, the result is a molecule of a compound.

230. A: Freezing point is the point at which a liquid changes to a solid.

231. D: The rate at which a chemical reaction occurs does not depend on the amount of mass lost, since the law of conservation of mass (or matter) states that in a chemical reaction there is no loss of mass.

232. B: Boyle's law states that for a constant mass and temperature, pressure and volume are related inversely to one another: $PV = c$, where c = constant.

233. C: An ionic bond forms when one atom donates an electron from its outer shell, called a valence electron, to another atom to form two oppositely charged atoms.

234. B: Metals are usually solids at room temperature, while nonmetals are usually gases at room temperature.

235. D: A solution that contains more hydroxide ions than hydrogen ions is a base, and bases have a pH greater than 7, so the only possible answer is D, 9.

236. B: Magnesium oxide cannot be found on the periodic table because it is a compound of two elements.

237. C: A solute is a substance that is dissolved in another substance. In this case, the solute is the spices.

238. B: Coulomb's law describes the electric force between two charged particles. It states that like charges repel and opposite charges attract, and the greater their distance, the less force they will exert on each other.

239. C: Conduction is the transfer of thermal energy between two substances that come into contact with each other; their particles must collide in order to transfer energy.

240. A: Solids contain the least amount of kinetic energy because they are made up of closely packed atoms or molecules that are locked in position and exhibit very little movement. Gases and plasmas exhibit the greatest amount of energy.

241. C: Vectors have a magnitude (e.g., 5 meters/second) and direction (e.g., towards north). Of the choice listed, only velocity has a direction. Speed, distance, and time are all quantities that have magnitude but not direction.

242. B: As you move from left to right across the periodic table, the atomic radius (size of the atom) decreases; it increases as you move down each group (from top to bottom). Electronegativity (the atom's ability to attract electrons), ionization energy (energy required to remove an electron from an atom), and electron affinity (the measure of energy changes with the addition of an electron) all generally increase as you move from left to right on the table. Moving down each group, electronegativity, ionization energy, and electron affinity all decrease.

243. A: Aluminum has a net charge of +3 (it's found in group 3 on the periodic table of elements). Hydroxide molecules are a group of atoms (hydrogen and oxygen) that have a net charge of -1. Therefore, you need three hydroxide groups are needed to balance the charge of the aluminum. The final molecular formula is $Al(OH)_3$.

244. B: According to Charles' law, temperature and volume are directly related. Avogadro's law describes how volume and the number of moles of a gas are related. The relationship between pressure and volume (they are inversely related) is expressed in Boyle's law. $PV = nRT$ is the ideal gas law and combines all of these variables in one master equation.

245. C: An alloy is a mixture of different elements and contains some of the properties of metals. Non-metals are found on the right side of the periodic table, while metals are found on the left. Network solids are exceptionally large and stable molecules with covalent bonds in multiple directions.

246. A: The process of sublimation occurs when a solid changes into a gas, while desublimation is the opposite process of changing a gas directly into a solid. Changing a liquid into a gas is called vaporization. Freezing is the name of the physical change from the liquid state to the solid state.

247. A: The pH of a solution is based on logarithmic relationships, specifically, powers of 10. This means that every point difference on the pH scale actually represents a tenfold change in the hydrogen ion concentration. If the pH decreases, the hydrogen ion concentration increases, and if the pH increases, hydrogen ion concentration decreases.

Anatomy and Physiology

248. A: HCG is secreted by the trophoblast, part of the early embryo, following implantation in the uterus. GnRH is secreted by the hypothalamus, while LH and FSH are secreted by the pituitary gland.

249. C: The layers are the tunica externa, tunica media, and tunica interna. Unlike most arteries, the pulmonary artery carries deoxygenated blood to the lungs for oxygenation. Blood flow in capillaries is significantly slower than in veins. Blood pressure is not always directly impacted by heart rate.

250. D: Skeletal, smooth, and cardiac are all types of muscle tissue. Adipose is not.

251. B: The only purpose of muscles is to produce movement through contraction

252. B: Anterior means toward the front of the body.

253. B: The brain is part of the nervous system.

254. B: Anatomy is the study of the structure and shape of the body.

255. A: Physiology is the study of how parts of the body function.

256. A: Circulation is transporting oxygen and other nutrients to the tissues via the cardiovascular system.

257. A: Smooth is not a type of connective tissue. Cartilage, adipose tissue, and blood tissue all are.

258. C: There are 11 organ systems in the human body.

259. B: The lymphatic system includes the spleen.

260. C: Proximal means close to the trunk of the body.

261. D: The lymphatic system, not the integumentary system, returns fluid to the blood vessels.

262. A: Optic refers to the eye or the way light is viewed.

263. A: Groups of cells that perform the same function are called tissues.

264. D: The nuclear division of somatic cells takes place during mitosis.

265. A: The immune system consists of the lymphatic system, spleen, tonsils, thymus and bone marrow.

266. A: A ribosome is a structure of eukaryotic cells that makes proteins.

267. A: Cortical bone is a connective tissue acting as a hard part of bones as organs. A liver is an organ, a mammal is a type of organism, and a hamstring is a muscle.

268. B: The adrenal glands are part of the endocrine system. They sit on the kidneys and produce hormones that regulate salt and water balance and influence blood pressure and heart rate.

269. B: Hemoglobin is a type of protein found in the red blood cells of all mammals.

270. D: Smooth muscle tissue involuntarily contracts to assist the digestive tract by moving the stomach and helping with the breakdown of food.

271. C: In respiration, food is used to produce energy as glucose and oxygen that react to produce carbon dioxide, water and ATP.

272. C: The pulmonary artery carries oxygen-depleted blood from the heart to the lungs. It is the last vessel the blood passes through before being re-oxygenated in the lungs.

Practice Test #2

Reading Comprehension

Questions 1–10 pertain to the following passage:

The disease known as rickets causes the bones to soften and creates a risk of bone fractures and even permanent bone deformation. It is most common in children, since their bones are already soft and are still growing. Rickets is believed to result from a lack of vitamin D and calcium, although some researchers will add a lack of phosphorus to this list. The disease is usually seen in parts of the world where children are suffering from poor nutrition. In the United States, doctors believed that the disease has been all but obsolete since the end of the Great Depression.

In fact, they were mistaken. Doctors are seeing a return of rickets, not just in the United States but also in other places where it was long since written off as no longer something to worry about. Cases of rickets are on the rise in states such as Georgia and North Carolina, and doctors are not entirely sure of the cause. They attribute the likely cause of the condition to poor nutrition and a lack of necessary vitamins and minerals. Many doctors believe that there is a twofold problem: low levels of calcium in young children who do not consume enough dairy products and low levels of vitamin D in breastfed babies. While breastfeeding is recommended, doctors point out that breast milk does not naturally contain high levels of vitamin D. This can be fine if the mother herself has adequate levels, but mothers with low levels of vitamin D will not provide enough for the baby as it nurses.

Among other developed nations, rickets is also making a reappearance in Great Britain. Doctors across England are seeing unexpected cases of rickets in children, and they believe that this is connected largely to low vitamin D levels. Some blame is placed on weather conditions, since Great Britain is not known for having copious amounts of sunshine, but also on lifestyle. Children are spending more time indoors watching television and playing video games, and in doing so they miss the sunshine when it is available. Additionally, parents are having their children wear sunscreen, which appears to be blocking what vitamin D would be absorbed while the children are outdoors.

Rickets is not yet considered an epidemic in developed nations, but there is enough concern among doctors and researchers to encourage awareness among parents. Children are encouraged to spend some time outdoors and to allow their skin to receive a little sun—just a few minutes a day is enough. Vitamin D and calcium supplements are also recommended, and nursing mothers are advised to have their levels checked. With any luck, rickets will once again become a disease of the past.

1. What is the author's primary purpose in writing the essay?

a. to persuade
b. to inform
c. to analyze
d. to entertain

2. What is the main idea of the passage?

a. Rickets should once again be a disease of the past
b. Rickets has once again become a problem in some developed nations
c. Children need vitamin D and calcium to avoid rickets, and nursing mothers need to have their levels checked
d. Rickets has reappeared only in the United States and Great Britain

3. Which of the following is *not* a detail from the passage?

a. A lack of phosphorus is a possible contributor to rickets
b. Sunscreen can block the skin's absorption of necessary vitamin D
c. Adults in Great Britain also have low vitamin D levels
d. Rickets has not been a problem in the United States since the time after the Great Depression

4. Based on the information provided in the passage, what can the reader infer about why the return of rickets is such a surprise in the United States?

a. The diet in the United States has improved since the Great Depression
b. People are already taking vitamin D and calcium supplements
c. Unlike in Great Britain, there is plenty of sunshine in many parts of the United States
d. Children in the United States spend enough time playing outdoors without wearing sunscreen

5. Which of the following *cannot* be inferred from the information in the passage?

a. Rickets has always been most common in third world nations among people who have a poor diet
b. Nursing mothers with low vitamin D levels should consider adding a supplement to their diet
c. The number of rickets cases in developed nations is not necessarily high, but the rise in expected cases is enough to concern doctors about the cause
d. Doctors are advising mothers with nursing babies to use formula that supplements vitamin D

6. Which of the following *can* be inferred from the information in the passage?

a. Doctors believe that the cases of rickets in Great Britain are linked more to lack of vitamin D than to low levels of calcium
b. Doctors now believe that children should not wear sunscreen while playing outside
c. Nursing mothers in Great Britain typically have higher levels of vitamin D in their breast milk
d. The majority of researchers believe that rickets is caused by lack of vitamin D and calcium only

7. The author uses the term *developed nations* to indicate which of the following in the passage?

a. nations that are constantly improving the status quo for citizens
b. nations that are world leaders in politics and economics
c. nations in which citizens receive plenty of sunshine for vitamin D absorption
d. nations in which most citizens have access to adequate nutritional options

8. What is the meaning of the word *copious* as it is used in the third paragraph?

a. abundant
b. small
c. expected
d. appropriate

9. What is the purpose of the final paragraph of the passage?

a. to offer solutions for preventing and eliminating rickets
b. to advise developing nations on how to avoid rickets
c. to warn nursing mothers about the importance of vitamin D
d. to provide hope for the future of a world without rickets

10. Which of the following is *not* a recommendation for ridding developed nations of rickets, as presented by the author?

a. People should consider taking vitamin D and calcium supplements
b. Children should get a little sun each day
c. Television and video games should be limited among children
d. Nursing mothers should have their vitamin D and calcium levels checked

Questions 11–20 pertain to the following passage:

So, your children got the chicken pox vaccine, and you think they will be all right. Not so fast. As it turns out, the chicken pox vaccine may only increase the risk of problems over time. Make no mistake: vaccination is not necessarily a bad thing, and vaccines have gone a long way toward eliminating illnesses that were once feared as life threatening or permanently disabling. But vaccines for some diseases, chicken pox in particular, come with side effects that create long-term uneasiness for doctors and researchers.

In fact, many scientists are increasingly concerned that *not* getting chicken pox might be more dangerous. Many people remember chicken pox as a standard childhood disease. Everyone seemed to get it, and everyone who had it probably knows that it is supposed to be a one-time deal. In others words, you catch chicken pox, scratch for about a week, and you never see it again—at least in theory. What happens in reality is that once a person catches chicken pox, the virus stays in the body. It typically remains dormant for the life of the individual, however, and the reason for this is only now being appreciated.

Researchers believe that those who have had chicken pox, those with the dormant virus in their bodies, should be around others who have had the disease. Doing so actually appears to boost the body's ongoing immunity against the virus. This means that spending time around children who have or have had chicken pox can help ensure that it never comes back. It can also help prevent the disease known as shingles later in life. Shingles, which is a more severe version of chicken pox, usually strikes adults after the age of sixty and can come with far more severe side effects than one week of scratching and sitting in an oatmeal bath. In some cases, shingles can cause problems that affect the sufferer for the rest of his or her life. But there appears to be a natural immunity that is built into getting chicken pox and then being around others with chicken pox, and researchers now believe that this explains the low rate of shingles that has traditionally been seen in the United States.

But what happens if very few people get chicken pox and most people are vaccinated? Children who are vaccinated do not contract the disease, and the amount of virus in the vaccine is not enough to boost immunity and thus prevent the contraction of shingles in many adults. And shingles is particularly dangerous because many of the elderly who contract it are already in poor health and struggle to recover from it. Some epidemiologists suggest that the use of the chicken pox vaccine in the United

States alone could lead to more than 20 million cases of shingles and at least 5,000 deaths from the disease. The potential concerns scientists enough that there remains ongoing debate about the value of the chicken pox vaccine.

11. What is the main idea of the passage?

a. Getting the chicken pox vaccine can lead to shingles later in life
b. Many children are getting the chicken pox vaccine throughout the United States
c. The chicken pox vaccine has the potential to create long-term problems
d. Chickenpox is no longer a childhood disease, as many adults now contract it

12. What is the author's primary purpose in writing the essay?

a. to entertain
b. to persuade
c. to analyze
d. to inform

13. Based on the information in the passage, what does an *epidemiologist* do?

a. study diseases among a population
b. study the internal organs of the human body
c. study viruses that are contracted among children
d. study adult problems that develop from childhood diseases

14. Which of the following is *not* a detail from the passage?

a. There are deaths from chicken pox each year in the United States
b. Shingles is a disease that develops from the same virus as chicken pox
c. Some researchers believe that not getting chicken pox can cause problems
d. Adults who contract shingles face a more dangerous disease than chicken pox

15. Based on the information in the passage, what is the value in contracting chicken pox during childhood?

a. to get it over with as early as possible
b. to avoid contracting shingles later in life
c. to have the dormant virus in the body throughout life
d. to demonstrate the body's natural immunity to some viruses

16. Based on the information in the passage, why is it important for people who have had chicken pox to be around others who have or have had the disease?

a. to help keep the disease in circulation and avoid shingles
b. to keep from catching chicken pox again
c. to boost the body's immunity to the virus
d. to maintain a low level of adult-contracted shingles

17. Which of the following *cannot* be inferred from the information in the passage?

a. People typically have contracted chicken pox in childhood
b. The age of shingles sufferers contributes to its serious effects on health
c. Many vaccines have helped rid society of dangerous diseases
d. Researchers believe that no one should get the chicken pox vaccine

18. Based on the information in the passage, why are some scientists concerned about extensive vaccination against chicken pox?

a. There is very little disease in the vaccine, but it is just enough for adults who have not had chicken pox to contract shingles
b. Researchers will be unable to locate enough subjects for ongoing study of health patterns among those who contract the disease
c. The contraction of chicken pox among adults is far more inconvenient than it is for children, so it is easier to contract the disease in childhood
d. Without frequent outbreaks of the disease, those who have already had it cannot build up their immunity to it

19. Which of the following pieces of information would make the author's point about the projected cases of shingles and deaths from shingles stronger in the final paragraph?

a. the names of researchers who are active in educating people about the chicken pox vaccine
b. the time period for the projected cases of shingles and the deaths from shingles
c. the countries where the chicken pox vaccine is currently in wide use
d. the number of people who are vaccinated against chicken pox each year

20. Which of the following *can* be inferred from the information in the final sentence?

a. More and more researchers are advising against widespread vaccination against chicken pox
b. The numbers are enough to concern researchers that the chicken pox vaccine might prove to do more harm than good
c. Researchers continue to evaluate and consider the long-term effects of the chicken pox vaccine
d. The concern about the effects of the chicken pox vaccine has led to a decrease in vaccinations

Questions 21–30 pertain to the following passage:

It seems like an obvious choice: do we destroy the final remaining samples of the smallpox virus or not? Smallpox, the terror that ravaged nations for centuries, was virtually destroyed in the latter part of the twentieth century—but not before it took about 500,000,000 people with it. Smallpox is one of the most dangerous viruses, attacking only humans (but not animals) and leaving only 70 percent of those infected with it alive. In some cases, survival brought its own challenges. The virus has been known to leave severe scarring, and many victims also lost their eyesight. Smallpox is so virulent that the small amount in the vaccine has been known to cause minor side effects.

So why would anyone want to keep samples around? Why not destroy what is left of the disease and eradicate it for good? After its successful inoculation program, the World Health Organization (WHO) has continued to maintain a selection of smallpox virus samples; more than 400 samples sit in laboratories in the United States and in Russia. The WHO has agreed that the samples should be consigned to the dustbin of history. They just cannot agree on whether all samples should be destroyed, and when the destruction should occur. The Soviet Union collapsed in 1991, but there were suggestions that the Soviet government, among others, had hidden samples of the smallpox virus separate from the official samples that were acknowledged. Should the WHO destroy all official samples, any remaining unofficial samples (never confirmed to be real) could be used to attack a population in an act of bioterrorism.

Without its own samples, the WHO and its researchers might be unable to create an effective treatment or vaccine.

Bioterrorism remains a real threat, and smallpox continues to be a concern for those looking at potential diseases that terrorists might use. What is more, the WHO points out that the majority of people today have no defense against outbreaks of the disease. Inoculation against smallpox ended in the early 1980s, and smallpox was declared to be officially defeated. Should a terrorist chose to attack people with smallpox, most would be completely susceptible to its dangers. As a result, many scientists—and particularly those who study infectious diseases—believe that the WHO should continue to delay destruction of the smallpox virus samples. Others claim that there are currently effective vaccines that could be used to protect a population. Even the two nations that hold these final samples are at loggerheads about the issue. One thing seems to be certain: the WHO still agrees that the smallpox samples should be destroyed. They just do not seem to know how *many* of the samples to destroy and *how soon*.

21. Which of the following words describes the author's primary purpose in writing the essay?

a. persuasive
b. Investigative
c. Expository
d. Advisory

22. What is the main idea of the passage?

a. The smallpox vaccine should be destroyed to eradicate the disease and prevent future outbreaks
b. The smallpox vaccine should not be destroyed to maintain samples that can be used in the event of a bioterrorism attack
c. The United States and Russia cannot agree on how many of the remaining smallpox samples to destroy, so the World Health Organization has stepped in to assist
d. The World Health Organization would prefer to destroy remaining samples of the smallpox vaccine but cannot decide when to do so

23. Which of the following is *not* a detail from the passage?

a. Smallpox killed at least half a billion people in the twentieth century alone
b. Samples of the smallpox virus are still kept in the Soviet Union
c. The smallpox virus has been known to cause both scarring and blindness
d. The World Health Organization instituted a smallpox vaccination program to eradicate the disease

24. Based on the information in the passage, what does the word *consigned* mean?

a. sent
b. refused
c. kept
d. hidden

25. Based on the information in the passage, why might the World Health Organization want to retain samples of the smallpox virus?

a. to develop a treatment and vaccine in the event of bioterrorism
b. to prevent acts of bioterrorism from those who hold secret samples of smallpox
c. to utilize the samples for continued research on the smallpox virus
d. to institute a new vaccination program that will protect people against future acts of bioterrorism

26. Which of the following *cannot* be inferred from the information in the passage?

a. The majority of people who contract the smallpox virus survive
b. The members of the World Health Organization are still trying to decide if all of the smallpox virus samples should be destroyed
c. The smallpox virus is one of the diseases that create concerns of bioterrorism for the World Health Organization
d. The World Health Organization is confident that there are secret samples of the smallpox virus being stored by terrorists

27. Based on the information in the passage, why do some researchers believe that it is now safe to destroy the remaining samples of the smallpox virus?

a. Because the disease is essentially obsolete, there is no need to maintain samples of it against future outbreaks
b. The collapse of the Soviet Union removed the risk of bioterrorism from the samples stored in that country and the United States
c. There is already a smallpox vaccine that could be used to protect people against outbreaks of the disease
d. Enough people have already been vaccinated against the smallpox virus and are protected against acts of bioterrorism

28. Since the World Health Organization was responsible for an inoculation program against smallpox, what can be inferred about the WHO's concern that the majority of people today are susceptible to the virus?

a. There are not enough people who are choosing to be vaccinated against smallpox
b. Very few are vaccinated today, and the vaccine has worn off for those who did receive it in the 1980s
c. The risks that accompany the smallpox vaccine have created concerns and have resulted in a reduction of vaccinations
d. Since smallpox is no longer seen as a threat, the majority of people do not believe that they are in any danger of contracting the virus

29. Based on the context of the passage, which of the following is the best definition for the expression *at loggerheads* in the final paragraph?

a. considering options
b. quietly discussing
c. eager to decide
d. in disagreement

30. Which of the following is *not* a detail from the passage?

a. The World Health Organization developed a widespread vaccination program and successfully combated the smallpox virus
b. While once considered a disease that only humans could contract, smallpox is slowly beginning to infect animals as well
c. Smallpox has been known to cause blindness in those who survive the disease
d. There are concerns that unofficial samples of the smallpox vaccine might have made it into the hands of governments other than that of the Soviet Union

Questions 31–37 pertain to the following passage:

The Black Death, a rapid and widespread outbreak of plague, first struck Europe in the fourteenth century. It also made several brief reappearances over the following centuries until it finally died off in the nineteenth century. Historians believe that the plague was responsible for the deaths of more than 50 percent of the population, killing between 75 million and 100 million people. The greatest fear of the Black Death was the sense of the unknown that it brought with it. The disease struck and spread quickly, and medieval doctors had no idea what caused it. (Today, many believe that rats were responsible for spreading the fleas that carried the disease. Oddly enough, many medieval people believed that it was the cats that were responsible and killed a large number of them, thus decreasing the opportunity to remove the real culprits.) Additionally, the plague killed some and not others—for no clear reason—and there was no known cure. Between 90 percent and 95 percent of those who contracted the disease died, and most within a week.

To understand the cause of such a devastating epidemic, scientists and historians have had to look back into history and piece together a puzzle. The majority accept the theory of the bubonic plague: rats carrying infected fleas made their way to various parts of Europe after arriving in the port cities, where the disease struck first. Some are not so sure, however. A few have argued that the flea-and-rat theory does not fit in with the symptoms, since fleas tend to attack the lower parts of the body, and it was the upper lymph nodes that showed the worse inflammation. Others point out that it would have been difficult for the fleas to stay alive long enough to infect people and spread the disease in Europe's cooler climate. One theory points to anthrax from cattle as a possible culprit, while another sees similarities between the spread of the Black Death and the spread of the Ebola virus. The exact cause(s) might never be known for certain. What is certain, though, is that the Black Death permanently changed Europe—and that no one wants to see it return.

31. Which of the following best describes the author's tone in the passage?

a. playful
b. concerned
c. definitive
d. explanatory

32. What is the main idea in the passage?

a. The Black Death had devastating effects in Europe, but scientists and historians are still not certain about what caused it
b. The spread of the Black Death suggests that the traditional theory about rats carrying infected fleas might not be accurate
c. The Black Death could have been prevented if medieval people had kept their cats alive instead of killing them
d. The Black Death was responsible for destroying more than half of Europe's population and is believed to have killed 100 million people

33. Which of the following is *not* a detail from the passage?

a. Europe continued to see outbreaks of the Black Death until the nineteenth century
b. Some scientists and historians have disagreed with the traditional view that infected fleas caused the Black Death
c. In addition to striking much of Europe, the Black Death also spread into parts of Asia
d. Medieval doctors were unsure of what caused the Black Death and could not treat it effectively

34. Which of the following *cannot* be inferred from the passage?

a. There might be more than one cause of the Black Death
b. The infection that caused the Black Death is related to the Ebola virus
c. While the death rate was high, some people survived the Black Death
d. The Black Death had far-reaching effects in Europe

35. Based on the information in the passage, why do some scientists and historians question the theory about the bubonic plague?

a. The symptoms of the Black Death and the climate of Europe appear to contradict the theory
b. The victims of the Black Death should have experienced inflammation in their lower lymph nodes
c. Current research suggests that the infection resembles anthrax more than bubonic plague
d. The fleas carrying the infection could not have lived long enough to create such a widespread epidemic

36. In the first paragraph, why does the author use parentheses around two of the sentences?

a. to create emphasis for the reader and indicate where the most important points are
b. to strengthen the main point by presenting important historical detail
c. to indicate interesting information that does not fit within the primary flow of thought
d. to include a supporting example from another source

37. Based on the information in the passage, which of the following can be assumed?

a. It is impossible to know for sure what caused the Black Death
b. The Ebola virus tends to spread quickly, just like the Black Death
c. Modern medicine has ensured that there will be no further outbreaks of the Black Death
d. Medieval doctors applied superstitious methods to treat outbreaks of the Black Death

Questions 38–42 pertain to the following passage:

It is a common summer ailment, and one that sends more than two million people to the doctor annually. It also tends to be a condition that most people forget about, until it is too late of course. Swimmer's ear might seem like a simple enough problem—a little water in the ear, a bit of swelling for a few days, some itching—but it affects millions of Americans annually and costs the medical industry at least $500 million per year. It can also create problems well beyond a few days of inconvenience. That is a lot for just a little water in the ear.

The problem, of course, is not the water itself but rather the quality of it and what happens when it remains in the ear canal. Swimming pools fill up during the summer months, and even the chlorine cannot keep the bacteria out. The bacteria that ends up floating in the water alongside swimmers can get into the ear canal, and when it does an infection can develop. Officially, this infection is known as otitis externa, but anyone who has experienced it knows it simply as swimmer's ear. With swimmer's ear, the ear canal becomes inflamed and, in extreme cases, can spread to the outside of the ear and even to parts of the face. In some, swimmer's ear has been known to cause temporary hearing loss.

The key to avoiding this condition is protecting the ears while around water and getting any water out as soon as possible. The longer that water remains in the ear canal, the better the chances that the bacteria will take up residence and cause an infection. If there is water in the ear, people are advised to avoid the old "head-banging" routine and utilize alcohol instead, as this pulls water out effectively without rattling the brain around. Doctors also advise using a soft towel to draw the water out, and some suggest using a blow dryer to remove the water.

38. What are the author's primary purposes in writing the essay?

a. to define and expand
b. to inform and advise
c. to present and persuade
d. to explain and approve

39. Which of the following *cannot* be inferred from the information in the passage?

a. Water in swimming pools can contain bacteria that causes infections in the ear canal
b. The infection that causes swimmer's ear leads to swelling in the ear canal
c. Swimmer's ear starts as a simple infection but can cause more serious problems
d. Anyone who gets water in his or her ear can expect to develop swimmer's ear

40. Which of the following is *not* a detail from the passage?

a. People can develop swimmer's ear from being in any body of water during the summer
b. The medical name for swimmer's ear is otitis externa
c. Swimmer's ear affects over one million people in the United States each year
d. Swimmer's ear results from bacteria in the water that gets into people's ear canals

41. Based on the information in the passage, why is swimmer's ear such a problem for people who spend time in swimming pools in the summer?

a. People shed body oils, skin, and bacteria when they use swimming pools, and these are a breeding ground for disease
b. Swimming pool maintenance crews cannot keep up with the increased activity in the pool during the hot summer months
c. The chlorine in the water is not sufficient to destroy the bacteria from such a large number of people in the pool
d. Swimmers do not use earplugs as much as they should, and this provides an opportunity for bacteria to get into the ear canal

42. Based on the information in the passage, which of the following is *not* a recommended course of action for removing water from the ear canal?

a. using alcohol to draw the water out
b. pressing a towel against the ear
c. shaking the head vigorously
d. drying the water with a blow dryer

Questions 43–47 pertain to the following passage:

It struck almost without warning: a headache, a chill, aching joints. A few hours later, the heat set in, and this led to intense sweating, dehydration, and delirium. Within a few more hours, death was expected to follow. The English of the fifteenth and sixteenth centuries were not sure what this disease was or what caused it; they only knew it as the "sweating sickness." Tens of thousands fell prey to it, and even though the numbers are not as high as some epidemics, the fear of the sweating sickness was greater due to the mystery surrounding it. Even today, the disease, not to mention its origin, has still not been identified. The sweating sickness disappeared from England in the 1570s, but the fact that no one is sure of what caused it leaves the door open for a possible return at some point.

Hygiene and sanitation are always the first culprits when searching for the source of an epidemic. Evils such as typhus and cholera are typically linked to filthy conditions in which disease can develop and spread. In general, these diseases tend to erupt first among the economically depressed who live in squalid conditions. But in the case of the sweating sickness, the disease seemed to have a magnetic attraction to the upper classes instead of the poor, and if anyone was more likely to be clean and have adequate sanitation, it was the wealthy.

Some scientists have suggested a bacterial fever, but the most likely results from the bites of lice and ticks. The English doctors who wrote about the disease made no mention of seeing such signs on victims. The latest theory points to the possibility of a hantavirus, which is a fast-acting disease that is carried by rodents and passed on when humans come in contact with them or their waste (however unintentionally). In the England of the fifteenth and sixteenth centuries, rodents were certainly a problem for rich and poor alike. But the problem with this theory is that humans cannot spread a hantavirus—as far as scientists know—but they almost certainly spread the sweating sickness. The cause of the sweating sickness might remain shrouded in mystery for now, but doctors and scientists continue research to make sure another epidemic does not occur in the future.

43. What is the main idea of the passage?

a. The sweating sickness was a mysterious illness that broke out in England in the fifteenth and sixteenth centuries, and scientists are still unsure about what caused it
b. The cause of the sweating sickness mystified fifteenth and sixteenth century doctors, but scientists today are beginning to solve the mystery of what caused the disease
c. The sweating sickness briefly attacked England in the fifteenth and sixteenth centuries, and it has not broken out anywhere since then
d. Modern-day scientists have narrowed the causes of sweating sickness down to a few options, but the lack of reporting from the fifteenth and sixteenth centuries make it impossible to confirm the cause

44. Which of the following is *not* a detail from the passage?

a. The sweating sickness struck quickly and often killed victims within a few hours
b. The sweating sickness is believed to have been caused by human contact with rodents and their waste
c. Doctors in the fifteenth and sixteenth centuries did not notice any strange bites that would suggest lice or ticks spread the sweating sickness
d. No cases of the sweating sickness have been seen in England since the latter part of the sixteenth century

45. Based on the information in the passage, which of the following can be inferred?

a. The sweating sickness was more likely to strike the wealthy instead of the poor in fifteenth and sixteenth century England
b. The sweating sickness is believed to have been spread from human contact
c. Other epidemics in England have resulted in far more deaths than the sweating sickness
d. The sweating sickness does not appear to have been caused by bad hygiene and sanitation among the poor

46. Based on the information in the passage, which of the following is known about hantaviruses?

a. Hantaviruses result from poor sanitary conditions and bad hygiene among the lower classes
b. Hantaviruses are carried by rodents and spread to humans through contact with rodents
c. Scientists now believe that some hantaviruses can be spread from contact between humans
d. The symptoms of the sweating sickness indicate that a hantavirus was the most likely cause

47. Based on the information in the passage, which of the following can be inferred about the sweating sickness?

a. Modern medical treatments mean that a return of the sweating sickness would not cause the same problems as it did in fifteenth and sixteenth century England
b. Doctors in fifteenth and sixteenth century England lacked the observational skills to notice any signs of bites from lice and ticks on patients
c. Because they do not know the cause, doctors and scientists are unsure about whether a new epidemic of sweating sickness will occur
d. The relatively low number of deaths from the sweating sickness suggests that many people in fifteenth and sixteenth century England did survive the disease

Vocabulary and General Knowledge

48. What is the meaning of the word *bifurcate*?

a. close
b. glow
c. split
d. speak

49. What is the best definition for the word *influx*?

a. acceptance
b. complexity
c. arrival
d. theory

50. What is the meaning of the word *substantiate*?

a. inhibit
b. assume
c. confirm
d. complete

51. What is the best definition for the word *typify*?

a. obscure
b. mock
c. announce
d. symbolize

52. What is the best definition for the word *sinuous*?

a. ominous
b. spoiled
c. supple
d. elaborate

53. What is the best definition for the word *transient*?

a. intermittent
b. temporary
c. hesitant
d. illusory

54. What is the best definition for the word *emaciated*?

a. vivid
b. fresh
c. grateful
d. wasted

55. What is the meaning of the word *irrevocable*?

a. binding
b. fortunate
c. unfeasible
d. indefinite

56. What is the meaning of the word *abate*?

a. enhance
b. remove
c. revive
d. reduce

57. What is the best definition for the word *extirpate*?

a. assist
b. define
c. provide
d. remove

58. What is the meaning of the word *feckless*?

a. incompetent
b. significant
c. relevant
d. headstrong

59. What is the meaning of the word *constrict*?

a. collect
b. appreciate
c. tighten
d. mingle

60. What is the meaning of the word *goad*?

a. create
b. force
c. bore
d. please

61. Select the meaning of the underlined word in this sentence:

With so much uncertainty about which decision was the best, the school provost submitted the various proposals to the board and ultimately chose the most <u>prevalent</u> favorite among the members.

a. dominant
b. old-fashioned
c. indifferent
d. scarce

62. What is the meaning of the word *nonchalant*?

a. excited
b. cowardly
c. unconcerned
d. imprudent

63. What is the best definition for the word *malinger*?

a. meet
b. prevent
c. pretend
d. surge

64. What is the meaning of the word *serrated*?

a. unusual
b. defiant
c. sad
d. jagged

65. What is the meaning of the word *contiguous*?

a. unique
b. adjacent
c. indirect
d. pleased

66. What is the meaning of the word *obfuscate*?

a. resemble
b. decide
c. conceal
d. surpass

67. What is the best definition for the word *portend*?

a. withdraw
b. deny
c. uncover
d. forecast

68. Select the best definition for the underlined word in this sentence:

> Although Nina was disappointed by the rude comment her supervisor made at the staff meeting, she decided to speak to him privately so he did not think she was trying to <u>undermine</u> him in front of everyone else.

a. disturb
b. encourage
c. challenge
d. present

69. What is the meaning of the word *immutable*?

a. unchangeable
b. breakable
c. desirable
d. flexible

70. What is the best definition for the word *protracted*?

a. required
b. extended
c. elevated
d. delayed

71. What is the best definition for the word *viable*?

a. inanimate
b. reasonable
c. likely
d. living

72. What is the best definition for the word *incessant*?

a. complicated
b. uncertain
c. constant
d. frightening

73. What is the meaning of the word *negligible*?

a. adequate
b. significant
c. minor
d. careless

74. What is the meaning of the word *accost*?

a. confront
b. insult
c. mock
d. evade

75. What is the meaning of the word *retreat*?

a. provide
b. contain
c. withdraw
d. anger

76. What is the meaning of the word *dichotomy*?

a. formation
b. decision
c. interruption
d. split

77. What is the best definition for the word *solicitous*?

a. plentiful
b. attentive
c. ignorant
d. stubborn

78. What is the best definition for the word *trajectory*?

a. direction
b. excitement
c. simplification
d. calculation

79. Select the meaning of the underlined word in this sentence:

The teacher took Agnes to task for her unwarranted comment about the new students in the class and how they were unable to afford better clothes.

a. justifiable
b. biased
c. essential
d. inappropriate

80. What is the meaning of the word *intemperate*?

a. unrestrained
b. unconcerned
c. idle
d. organized

81. What is the meaning of the word *onerous*?

a. trivial
b. motivating
c. demanding
d. urgent

82. What is the meaning of the word *heterogeneous*?

a. different
b. unusual
c. clear
d. comparable

83. What is the best definition for the word *overwrought*?

a. agitated
b. respected
c. indifferent
d. excessive

84. What is the best definition for the word *dotage*?

a. strength
b. senility
c. balance
d. position

85. What is the best definition for the word *puerile*?

a. youthful
b. sophisticated
c. virtuous
d. childish

86. What is the meaning of the word *putative*?

a. chosen
b. factual
c. accepted
d. affective

87. What is the meaning of the word *enumerate*?

a. refuse
b. plead
c. include
d. specify

88. What is the best definition for the word *intangible*?

a. sudden
b. vague
c. forthright
d. definite

89. What is the meaning of the word *relapse*?

a. prevention
b. endearment
c. progression
d. setback

90. What is the best definition for the word *definitive*?

a. absurd
b. incomplete
c. ultimate
d. preferred

91. What is the meaning of the word *conflate*?

a. falsify
b. merge
c. anticipate
d. expand

92. What is the best definition for the word *congenital*?

a. contracted
b. lifelong
c. additional
d. innate

93. What is the best definition for the word *gestate*?

a. conceive
b. provide
c. delete
d. remind

94. What is the meaning of the word *mordant*?

a. elegant
b. soothing
c. joking
d. disrespectful

95. What is the meaning of the word *transmute*?

a. annoy
b. maintain
c. change
d. charge

96. What is the meaning of the word *circumscribe*?

a. continue
b. enclose
c. converse
d. permit

97. What is the best definition for the word *prehensile*?

a. gentle
b. clever
c. greedy
d. gracious

Grammar

98. Select the combination of words that makes the following sentence grammatically correct.

Detective Melchior tried to ___________ the solution by winking vigorously, but his sidekick was unable to __________ the detective's meaning and asked, "Why are you winking, sir?"

a. infer, imply
b. imply, infer
c. imply, imply
d. infer, infer

99. Select the following sentence that is in the *active tense*.

a. The child was given presents by his friends for his birthday
b. The winner of the marathon was rewarded with a medal by the awards committee
c. The fashion designer presented his newest collection on the Paris runways
d. The aromatic duck a l'orange was quickly devoured by the eager culinary students

100. Select the combination of words that makes the following sentence grammatically correct.

___________ of my time is spent in completing the ___________ tasks that I have each day.

a. many, much
b. many, many
c. much, many
d. much, much

101. Select the combination of words that makes the following sentence grammatically correct.

Because Edwina had _________ time than she expected, she ran to the express lane in the grocery store, despite the fact that she had more than the required "Ten Items or _________."

a. fewer, fewer
b. fewer, less
c. less, less
d. less, fewer

102. Select the word or phrase that is correctly capitalized for the following sentence.

The eighth-grade students recently completed their study of the Battle of Verdun during ___________.

a. world war I
b. World War I
c. World war i
d. World war I

103. Select the word or phrase that is correctly capitalized for the following sentence.

Historians have traditionally believed that more than one million people died during the ____________, but some argue that the figure should be revised to upward of four million.

a. siege of Leningrad
b. siege Of Leningrad
c. Siege of Leningrad
d. siege of leningrad

104. Select the word or phrase that is correctly capitalized for the following sentence.

Leo's planetary studies led him to review Saturn, Neptune, Jupiter, ____________.

a. Earth, and the Sun
b. earth, and the Sun
c. Earth, and the sun
d. earth, and the sun

105. Select the word or phrase that is correctly abbreviated for the following sentence.

The doctor wrote out the details of the prescription, noting the specific amount of milligrams that the patient needed to take: "________ to be taken each day."

a. 4 mlg
b. 4 mgr
c. 4 m
d. 4 mg

106. Select the word or phrase that makes the following sentence grammatically correct.

My two friends, Janet and ________, are planning to join us at the opera this weekend.

a. she
b. her
c. they
d. them

107. Select the word or phrase that makes the following sentence grammatically correct.

Emily noticed that the book was not sitting where she had left it, and she shrieked, "Somebody ________ been in my house!"

a. have
b. will
c. has
d. might

108. Select the word or phrase that makes the following sentence grammatically correct.

The head of the student council noted, "With the increase in tuition prices, the financial burden placed on ____________ guarantees that we will be expected to pay far more than we can reasonably afford."

a. those students
b. we students
c. us students
d. them students

109. Select the word or phrase that makes the following sentence grammatically correct.

The new benefit plan applies to ____________ employees in the agency.

a. part- and full-time
b. part and full-time
c. part and full time
d. part/ and full/time

110. Select the combination of words that makes the following sentence grammatically correct.

_________ that foul-smelling cup of tea away, and ________ me something that I can actually drink.

a. bring, take
b. bring, bring
c. take, bring
d. take, take

111. Select the word or phrase that makes the following sentence grammatically correct.

You ____________ to get your oil changed before you damage your vehicle.

a. ought
b. had ought
c. should ought
d. had

112. Select the word or phrase that makes the following sentence grammatically correct.

Dr. Watson shook his head in bemusement at ____________ explanation of his deductive reasoning skills.

a. Sherlock Holmes'
b. Sherlock Holme's
c. Sherlock Holmes's
d. Sherlock Holmes

113. Select the word or phrase that makes the following sentence grammatically correct.

The detective novel was so well written that Linus was completely shocked by the __________ solution.

a. mysteries
b. mystery's
c. mysteries'
d. mysterie's

114. Select the word or phrase that makes the following sentence grammatically correct.

Both Hugo and Camille ________ members of their local rotary club and frequently participate in the annual auction to raise money for charity.

a. is
b. was
c. were
d. are

115. Select the combination of words that makes the following sentence grammatically correct.

The coach tried to motivate his team by saying, "This year we will _________ to the challenge and ___________ the bar for what we can accomplish together."

a. rise, raise
b. raise, raise
c. raise, rise
d. rise, rise

116. Select the combination of words that makes the following sentence grammatically correct.

Do not _________ down just yet; I need to _________ new sheets on that bed.

a. lay, lay
b. lay, lie
c. lie, lie
d. lie, lay

117. Select the combination of words that makes the following sentence grammatically correct.

__________ car has broken down, so __________ going to go to Evan's house and stay ___________ until the car is repaired.

a. their, they're, there
b. they're, their, they're
c. there, they're, their
d. there, their, there

118. Select the combination of words that makes the following sentence grammatically correct.

____________ the two of us, I don't think there's much intelligence _________ all ten of the board members.

a. among, among
b. among, between
c. between, among
d. between, between

119. Select the punctuation that makes the following sentence grammatically correct.

a. The committee will discuss the different options for the new park at the following meetings March 19th and March 26th.
b. The committee will discuss the different options for the new park at the following meetings; March 19th and March 26th.
c. The committee will discuss the different options for the new park at the following meetings: March 19th and March 26th.
d. The committee will discuss the different options for the new park at the following meetings, March 19th and March 26th.

120. Select the punctuation that makes the following sentence grammatically correct.

a. Margot's business travels have taken her to Topeka Kansas El Paso Texas and San Diego California.
b. Margot's business travels have taken her to Topeka, Kansas, El Paso, Texas, and San Diego, California.
c. Margot's business travels have taken her to Topeka Kansas, El Paso Texas, and San Diego California.
d. Margot's business travels have taken her to Topeka, Kansas; El Paso, Texas; and San Diego, California.

121. Select the punctuation that makes the following sentence grammatically correct.

a. Honestly, Mateo what you're suggesting is impossible.
b. Honestly Mateo; what you're suggesting is impossible.
c. Honestly. Mateo: what you're suggesting is impossible.
d. Honestly, Mateo, what you're suggesting is impossible.

122. Select the combination of words that makes the following sentence grammatically correct.

__________ Marine, no one else wanted to go with Elsa and get some sun __________ the pool.

a. beside, besides
b. besides, beside
c. beside, beside
d. besides, besides

123. Select the punctuation that makes the following sentence grammatically correct.

a. The more time we have to complete the project the better we will be.
b. The more time we have to complete the project; the better we will be.
c. The more time we have to complete the project: the better we will be.
d. The more time we have to complete the project, the better we will be.

124. Select the punctuation that makes the following sentence grammatically correct.

a. Jeannette, the guests will be arriving at what time
b. Jeannette, the guests will be arriving at what time?
c. Jeannette, the guests will be arriving at what time...
d. Jeannette, the guests will be arriving at what time.

125. Select the word or phrase that makes the following sentence grammatically correct.

Either Eleanor or Patrick __________ given the job of picking up the ice for the party.

a. should
b. are
c. was
d. were

126. Select the word or phrase that makes the following sentence grammatically correct.

Edgar ______________ to be there, but the trains were delayed by several hours.

a. had liked
b. would like
c. was liking
d. would have liked

127. Select the word or phrase that makes the following sentence grammatically correct.

If I ___________ more diligent, I would tackle my housework in a more timely manner.

a. were
b. are
c. am
d. was

128. Select the word or phrase that makes the following sentence grammatically correct.

She insisted that the children __________ inside the house no later than four o'clock.

a. will be
b. be
c. are
d. were

129. Select the word or phrase that makes the following sentence grammatically correct.

The car needs ____________ before we leave for our road trip.

a. cleaned
b. to clean
c. cleaning
d. to be cleaned

130. Select the word or phrase that makes the following sentence grammatically correct.

Knowing the impending danger, he went forward _____________ and with great care.

a. cautiously
b. caution
c. cautious
d. cautioned

131. Select the word or phrase that makes the following sentence grammatically correct.

She assured the doctor that she felt __________ enough to take the vacation that she had been planning.

a. good
b. better
c. well
d. best

132. Select the word or phrase that makes the following sentence grammatically correct.

The town's one-hundred-year anniversary was a ______________ event; even the state governor showed up to shake a few hands and congratulate the residents.

a. important
b. real important
c. really important
d. more important

133. Select the word or phrase that makes the following sentence grammatically correct.

Cedric was feeling weak because he ______________ food all day.

a. had any
b. barely had any
c. had barely no
d. had barely any

134. Select the combination of words that makes the following sentence grammatically correct.

Meg was ______________ than Beth and Jo, but Amy was considered to be the ______________ of the four March girls.

a. prettier, prettier
b. prettier, prettiest
c. prettiest, prettier
d. prettiest, prettiest

135. Select the word or phrase that makes the following sentence grammatically correct.

For Thomas, seeing the live concert at the stadium was ______________ and life-changing experience.

a. the most unique
b. a unique
c. the uniquest
d. a more unique

136. Select the combination of words that makes the following sentence grammatically correct.

He refused to consider ______________ which route to the store would be best so he would not go ______________ than necessary.

a. farther, further
b. farther, farther
c. further, further
d. further, farther

137. Select the combination of words that makes the following sentence grammatically correct.

Zenaida felt ___________ that the child was doing so ___________ in the math class.

a. bad, bad
b. badly, bad
c. bad, badly
d. badly, badly

138. Select the combination of words that makes the following sentence grammatically correct.

Jerome put the matter to the ___________ for the consideration, assured that they would offer the ___________ he so desperately needed.

a. council, counsel
b. council, council
c. counsel, counsel
d. counsel, council

139. Select the combination of words that makes the following sentence grammatically correct.

Please ___________ me on the best choice for a contractor; I have so many options, and I am in need of sound ___________.

a. advise, advice
b. advice, advise
c. advice, advice
d. advise, advise

140. Select the combination of words that makes the following sentence grammatically correct.

Our true emotions can often ___________ us. That's what the poet was trying to ___________ to in the romantic ballad.

a. allude, allude
b. elude, elude
c. allude, elude
d. elude, allude

141. Select the word or phrase that makes the following sentence grammatically correct.

Because Carl's truck broke down, he had to take four different ___________ to get to work.

a. busses
b. buses
c. bus
d. bus's

142. Select the punctuation that makes the following sentence grammatically correct.

a. The professor lectured on Pushkin: Today most scholars recognize that The Bronze Horseman both reveres Peter the Great and calls into question his tyrannical behavior.
b. The professor lectured on Pushkin: "Today most scholars recognize that the poem *The Bronze Horseman* both reveres Peter the Great and calls into question his tyrannical behavior."
c. The professor lectured on Pushkin: "Today most scholars recognize that the poem "*The Bronze Horseman*" both reveres Peter the Great and calls into question his tyrannical behavior."
d. The professor lectured on Pushkin: "Today most scholars recognize that the poem "The Bronze Horseman" both reveres Peter the Great and calls into question his tyrannical behavior".

143. Which word is *not* spelled correctly in the context of the following sentence?

When they hurried the magnificent conveyance along, they were sure that they would be victoryous.

a. hurried
b. magnificent
c. conveyance
d. victoryous

144. Which word is *not* spelled correctly in the context of the following sentence?

Professor Rinkie told the story but preferred omitting the forgettable occurence with the horses.

a. preferred
b. omitting
c. forgettable
d. occurence

145. Choose the word or words that best fill the blank.

Marty did not realize until he arrived to perform in Philadelphia that he had left his guitar in Pittsburgh; ______, he was fortunate to find a music store that agreed to rent him one for the evening.

a. however
b. because
c. after
d. while

146. Choose the sentence that is correct and most clearly written.

a. The novelist David Markson is known for his experimental works, such as "This Is Not a Novel."
b. Experimental works such as "This Is Not a Novel" have been wrote by David Markson.
c. Novelist David Markson is knew for his experimental works, such as "This Is Not a Novel."
d. David Markson is a novelist who is known for experimentation his works include "This Is Not a Novel."

147. Choose the sentence that is correct and most clearly written.

a. I intended to mow the yard, but I wanted to wait until evening when it are cooler.
b. I intended to mow the yard, but I wanted to wait until evening when it would be cooler.
c. I intended to mow the yard, but not until it getting cooler in the evening.
d. I intended to mow the yard, but I waits until evening when it was cooler.

Mathematics

148. What number is 75% of 500?

a. 365
b. 375
c. 387
d. 390

149. $(\mathbf{7} \times \mathbf{5}) + (\mathbf{8} \times \mathbf{2}) = ?$

a. 51
b. 57
c. 85
d. 560

150. $(\mathbf{8} \div \mathbf{2}) \times (\mathbf{12} \div \mathbf{3}) = ?$

a. 1
b. 8
c. 12
d. 16

151. Which of the following numbers is a factor of 36?

a. 5
b. 7
c. 8
d. 9

152. $\mathbf{75} \times \mathbf{34} = ?$

a. 1200
b. 2050
c. 2550
d. 3100

153. Solve for *x*:

$$x + 372 = 853$$

a. 455
b. 481
c. 520
d. 635

154. Which fraction is equivalent to the decimal 0.25?

a. $\frac{1}{4}$
b. $\frac{1}{2}$
c. $\frac{1}{8}$
d. $\frac{2}{3}$

155. The decimal 0.85 is equivalent to which fraction?

a. $\frac{13}{15}$
b. $\frac{17}{20}$
c. $\frac{18}{19}$
d. $\frac{19}{22}$

156. Which of the following fractions is closest to $\frac{2}{3}$ without going over?

a. $\frac{6}{13}$
b. $\frac{7}{12}$
c. $\frac{11}{16}$
d. $\frac{9}{12}$

157. A circle graph is used to show the percentage of each patient class that a hospital sees. If $\frac{1}{3}$ of the patients seen are pediatric patients, how much of the circle should indicate pediatric?

a. 90 degrees
b. 120 degrees
c. 180 degrees
d. 210 degrees

158. A traveler spent $25 on food during his first week of vacation. He then spent $52 on food each of the next two weeks. The fourth week he spent $34 on food. What was his average weekly food expenditure over his four-week vacation?

a. $ 37.00
b. $ 38.25
c. $ 40.75
d. $ 52.00

159. $437.65 - 325.752 = ?$

a. 111.898
b. 121.758
c. 122.348
d. 133.053

160. $43.3 \times 23.03 = ?$

a. 997.199
b. 999.999
c. 1010.03
d. 1111.01

161. After two weeks of dieting, a patient lost 6% of their original body weight. If the original weight was 157 pounds, what was the final weight after two weeks (to the nearest pound)?

a. 139 lbs
b. 142 lbs
c. 145 lbs
d. 148 lbs

162. In order for a school to allow a vending machine to be placed next to the cafeteria, 65% of the student population must request it. If 340 of the school's 650 students have already requested the vending machine, how many more must request it in order for the vending machine to be installed?

a. 75
b. 83
c. 89
d. 99

163. Round this number to the nearest hundredth: 390.24657

a. 400
b. 390.247
c. 390.25
d. 390.2

164. What number, when multiplied by $\frac{4}{5}$, gives an answer of 1?

a. $\frac{5}{4}$
b. $\frac{1}{2}$
c. $\frac{1}{4}$
d. $\frac{4}{3}$

165. During a given week, a patient's sodium intake was 300 mg on Monday, 1240 mg on Tuesday, 900 mg on Wednesday and on Friday, and 1500 mg on Thursday. What was the patient's average sodium intake for those five days?

a. 476 mg
b. 754 mg
c. 968 mg
d. 998 mg

166. Which of the following numbers is correctly rounded to the nearest tenth?

a. 3.756 rounds to 3.76
b. 4.567 rounds to 4.5
c. 6.982 rounds to 7.0
d. 54.32 rounds to 54.4

167. Which of the following fractions is equivalent to the decimal 0.625?

a. 3/4
b. 5/6
c. 5/8
d. 2/3

168. A 6% (by volume) solution of bleach in water is required for cleaning a bathroom. How many mL of the solution can be made from 50 mL of pure bleach?

a. 833 mL
b. 952 mL
c. 1054 mL
d. 2000 mL

169. $\mathbf{8.7 \times 23.3} = ?$

a. 202.71
b. 2027.1
c. 212.71
d. 2127.1

170. $\mathbf{134.5 \div 5} = ?$

a. 26.9
b. 25.9
c. 23.9
d. 22.9

171. $\mathbf{23 \div 3} = ?$

a. $6\frac{2}{3}$
b. $7\frac{1}{3}$
c. $7\frac{2}{3}$
d. $8\frac{1}{3}$

172. $\mathbf{4500 + 3422 + 3909} = ?$

a. 12,831
b. 12,731
c. 11,831
d. 11,731

173. $\mathbf{14,634 + 7,377} = ?$

a. 21,901
b. 21,911
c. 22,011
d. 22,901

174. $\mathbf{9,645 - 6,132} = ?$

a. 2,513
b. 2,517
c. 3,412
d. 3,513

175. $\mathbf{893 \times 64} = ?$

a. 54,142
b. 56,822
c. 56,920
d. 57,152

176. $\mathbf{29,294 \div 97} = ?$

a. 302
b. 322
c. 3002
d. 3022

177. What is the decimal equivalent of $\frac{38}{100}$?

a. 3.8
b. 0.38
c. 0.038
d. 0.0038

178. $\mathbf{6.8 + 11.3 + 0.06} = ?$

a. 17.16
b. 17.70
c. 18.16
d. 18.70

179. $\mathbf{0.28 \times 0.17} = ?$

a. 0.226
b. 0.476
c. 0.0226
d. 0.0476

180. Which numeral is in the thousandths place in 0.3874?

a. 3
b. 8
c. 7
d. 4

181. What is the equivalent decimal number for five hundred twelve thousandths?

a. 0.512
b. 0.0512
c. 512,000
d. 0.00512

182. $\mathbf{3\frac{1}{8} + 6 + \frac{3}{7}} = ?$

a. $9\frac{31}{56}$
b. $9\frac{1}{2}$
c. $9\frac{21}{56}$
d. $9\frac{7}{8}$

183. $\mathbf{4\frac{1}{7} - 2\frac{1}{2}} = ?$

a. $2\frac{5}{14}$
b. $1\frac{5}{14}$
c. $1\frac{9}{14}$
d. $2\frac{9}{14}$

184. $\mathbf{1\frac{1}{4}} \times \mathbf{3\frac{2}{5}} \times \mathbf{1\frac{2}{3}} = ?$

a. $7\frac{1}{12}$
b. $5\frac{5}{6}$
c. $6\frac{7}{12}$
d. $8\frac{11}{15}$

185. $\mathbf{\frac{3}{5}} \div \mathbf{\frac{1}{2}} = ?$

a. $1\frac{1}{5}$
b. $\frac{3}{10}$
c. $1\frac{7}{10}$
d. $\frac{4}{5}$

186. Which of the following equations is true?

a. $\frac{4}{7} = \frac{12}{21}$
b. $\frac{3}{4} = \frac{12}{20}$
c. $\frac{5}{8} = \frac{15}{32}$
d. $\frac{7}{9} = \frac{28}{35}$

187. Solve for *n* in the following equation:

$$\frac{n}{7} = \frac{18}{21}$$

a. 3
b. 4
c. 5
d. 6

188. Reduce $\mathbf{\frac{14}{98}}$ to the lowest possible terms.

a. $\frac{7}{49}$
b. $\frac{2}{14}$
c. $\frac{1}{7}$
d. $\frac{3}{8}$

189. Express $\frac{68}{7}$ as a mixed number.

a. $9\frac{5}{7}$
b. $8\frac{4}{7}$
c. $9\frac{3}{7}$
d. $8\frac{6}{7}$

190. What percentage is equivalent to thirty-six hundredths?

a. 36%
b. 0.36%
c. 0.036%
d. 3.6%

191. What percentage of 60 is the number 3?

a. 5%
b. 9%
c. 15%
d. 20%

192. What percentage of 25 is the number 1?

a. 1%
b. 2%
c. 3%
d. 4%

193. What number is three eighths of 40?

a. 15
b. 20
c. 22
d. 24

194. What percentage of $\frac{5}{6}$ is the fraction $\frac{1}{3}$?

a. 10%
b. 20%
c. 30%
d. 40%

195. What percentage is equivalent to a 3:15 part-to-whole ratio?

a. 5%
b. 0.5%
c. 2%
d. 20%

196. What percentage is equivalent to the fraction $\frac{3}{12}$?

a. 0.25%
b. 0.04%
c. 25%
d. 40%

197. What is the most simplified fractional equivalent to 8%?

a. $\frac{2}{50}$
b. $\frac{4}{5}$
c. $\frac{2}{5}$
d. $\frac{2}{25}$

Biology

198. Which chemicals are responsible for conveying an impulse along a nerve cell?

a. Sodium and potassium
b. Calcium
c. Actin and myosin
d. Phosphorus

199. What type of genetic mutation occurs when a piece of DNA breaks off the chromosome and attaches to a different chromosome?

a. Nondisjunction
b. Translocation
c. Deletion
d. Crossing over

200. What is the first line of defense against invading bacteria?

a. The skin
b. Macrophages
c. T-cells
d. Lymphocytes

201. What is the purpose of capping the 5' end of mRNA?

a. To signal the end of the mRNA strand
b. To prepare it to attach to the complementary DNA strand
c. To protect the end of the strand from degradation
d. There is no known reason for capping the end of an mRNA strand

202. During what process does hydrolysis occur to provide electrons to chlorophyll, which subsequently absorb energy?

a. Light-dependent reactions of photosynthesis
b. Light-independent reactions of photosynthesis
c. Calvin cycle
d. Krebs cycle

203. What is the process called when root hairs capture water and move it upwards into the rest of the plant?

a. Photosynthesis
b. Diffusion
c. Active transport
d. Transpiration

204. Which plant hormone causes fruit to ripen?

a. Auxins
b. Cytokinins
c. Ethylene
d. Abscisic Acid

205. What is thigmotropism?

a. Growth of plant materials toward light
b. Growth of leaves and stems opposite to the pull of gravity
c. Growth toward a source of nutrition
d. Growth of plant structures in response to contact with a physical structure

206. What is the purpose of the stigma?

a. To gather pollen
b. To attract pollinators like birds and bees
c. To nourish the fertilized ovum
d. To produce pollen

207. Organisms with the same _________ are most closely related.

a. order
b. genus
c. family
d. class

208. What are the first life forms to colonize a new area called?

a. Primary producers
b. Pioneer species
c. Primary consumers
d. Primary succession

209. Which of the following fibers is not found in the cytoskeleton?

a. Microtubules
b. Microfilaments
c. Glycoproteins
d. Intermediate filaments

210. Which biome is characterized by a population of cone-bearing trees?

a. Tropical forest
b. Tundra
c. Temperate deciduous forest
d. Coniferous forest

211. Which of the following is an example of an abiotic factor?

a. Local vegetation
b. Sunlight
c. Endemic populations
d. Ecosystem

212. Detritivores eat only what type of matter?

a. Plants
b. Animals
c. Both plants and animals
d. Dead and decaying matter

213. What type of population curve is produced once exponential growth is leveling off?

a. S-curve
b. J-curve
c. K-curve
d. R-curve

214. When one partner benefits and the other is harmed, what symbiotic relationship is formed?

a. Mutualism
b. Commensalism
c. Parasitism
d. Predation

215. In mice, brown fur is the dominant trait, and the recessive trait is white fur. In a cross between two heterozygous mice, how many offspring will be white if 24 mice result from the cross?

a. 6
b. 12
c. 18
d. 24

216. You are crossing fruit flies with two distinct traits: eye color and the presence/absence of wings. Having red eyes and the presence of wings are both dominant traits, while the recessive phenotypes are white eyes and the absence of wings. If you are crossing two flies that are heterozygous for both traits, what fraction of flies would you expect to have wings and white eyes?

a. 0/16
b. 1/16
c. 3/16
d. 9/16

217. Which of the following is true about sex-linked traits?

a. They never occur in females
b. They occur rarely in females
c. The trait appears on the Y chromosome
d. Sons usually inherit the trait from their father

218. Which of the following is not found on the exterior of most prokaryotic cells?

a. Pili
b. Flagella
c. Capsule
d. Plasma membrane

219. Which of the following will affect enzymatic activity?

a. Temperature
b. Amount of water
c. Form of the enzyme
d. Concentration of fatty acids

220. Transcription of the genetic material occurs when:

a. DNA is copied identically to be distributed to its daughter cells
b. DNA is copied into the complementary form of mRNA
c. DNA is converted to the coded protein
d. the message is edited into a form that the ribosome can understand

221. Where does translation occur?

a. In the nucleus
b. In the centrosome
c. In the ribosome
d. In the cytoplasm

222. What type of selection is occurring when the intermediate trait, not either of the extremes, is the driving force?

a. Divergent Evolution
b. Disruptive Evolution
c. Directional Selection
d. Stabilizing Selection

Chemistry

223. The concentration of hydrogen ions in a neutral solution is:

a. 7
b. 10^{7}
c. 10^{-7}
d. 10^{-14}

224. What will adding an acid to a base will yield?

a. A neutral solution
b. A salt
c. An acid
d. A base

225. Alcohols have which common structure?

a. A benzene ring
b. A carbon atom with a double bond to an oxygen atom and a single bond to a hydroxyl group
c. A nitrogen bond which is also bonded to other carbon atoms
d. A hydroxyl group

226. Which of the following is an example of a primary amine?

a. 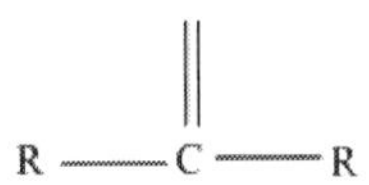

b. 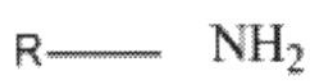

c. 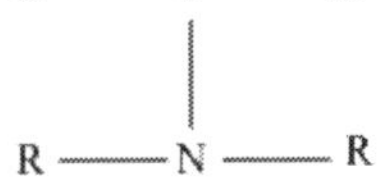

d. 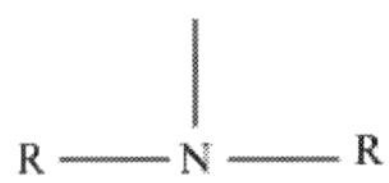

227. Which of the following is not true of hydrocarbons?

a. They are volatile
b. They have low boiling points
c. Nonpolar/London dispersion forces hold the hydrocarbon together
d. Most hydrocarbons are solids

228. What is the primary difference between ketones and aldehydes?

a. Ketones contain two functional groups and a double-bonded oxygen attached to a central carbon atom, while aldehydes contain only one functional group, a hydrogen atom, and a double-bonded oxygen atom bonded to the central carbon.
b. Aldehydes contain two functional groups and a double-bonded oxygen attached to a central carbon atom, while ketones contain only one functional group, a hydrogen atom, and a double-bonded oxygen atom bonded to the central carbon.
c. Ketones are polar substances, and aldehydes are nonpolar substances.
d. Aldehydes are polar substances, and ketones are nonpolar substances.

229. What type of organic reaction occurs when water is released as two functional groups bond together?

a. Substitution
b. Hydrolysis
c. Condensation
d. Radical reaction

230. Which of the following is the Lewis Dot structure for NO_3^-?

a. 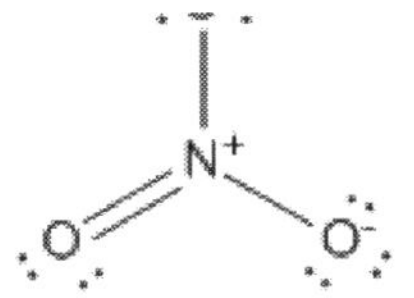

b. 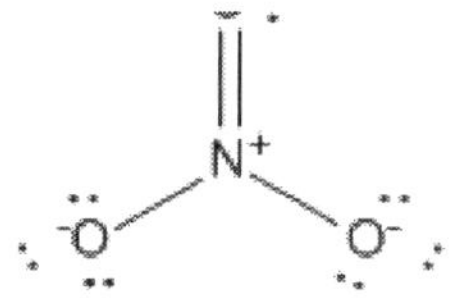

c. 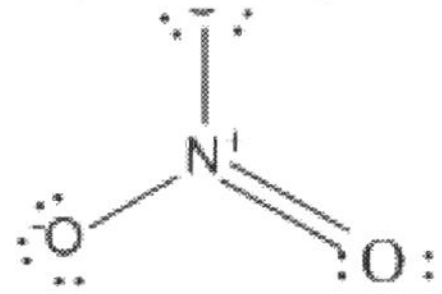

d. All of the above

231. What is the release of a massive amount of energy caused by the bombarding and splitting of a nucleus by a neutron called?

a. Positron emission
b. Nuclear fission
c. Controlled fusion
d. Electron capture

232. How many valence electrons do the noble gases contain in their valence shell?

a. 2
b. 4
c. 6
d. 8

233. What is one mole equal to?

a. 6.02×10^{23} units
b. 6.02×10^{-23} units
c. 6.02×10^{10} units
d. 6.02×10^{-10} units

234. A patient has a temperature of 99.1 degrees Fahrenheit. What is the temperature in Kelvin?

a. 372 Kelvin
b. 310 Kelvin
c. 273 Kelvin
d. 37.3 Kelvin

235. A sample of O_2 gas is heated from 35°C to 100°C. The final pressure of the gas is 2.5 atm. What was the initial pressure of the gas if the volume of the container remained constant through the heating process?

a. 0.875 atm
b. 2.1 atm
c. 7.1 atm
d. 10 atm

236. Increasing the volume of a gas will:

a. decrease the temperature.
b. increase the number of moles of the gas.
c. decrease the pressure of the gas.
d. make the gas more volatile.

237. A covalent bond occurs when:

a. two atoms bond together
b. one electron transfers from one atom to another, forming two ions
c. both bonding electrons come from the same atom
d. an electron pair is shared between two atoms, creating the bond

238. Which of the following is released during a combustion reaction?

a. Water
b. Heat
c. Oxygen
d. Electrons

239. Which of the following is an example of a colligative property?

a. Boiling point depression
b. Freezing point elevation
c. Freezing point depression
d. Elevation of vapor pressure

240. After balancing the following reaction, what is the coefficient of the molecule of water?

$C_6H_{12}O_6 + O_2 \rightarrow CO_2 + H_2O$

a. 1
b. 2
c. 3
d. 6

241. According to the second law of thermodynamics:

a. energy is neither created nor destroyed
b. entropy is always increasing in the universe
c. the entropy of a crystal at absolute zero temperature is zero
d. enthalpy increases within a universe

242. When two atoms are triple bonded to each other, how many electrons do they share?

a. 1
b. 2
c. 3
d. 6

243. Hydrophobic molecules are:

a. nonpolar
b. polar
c. dipolar
d. unipolar

244. Which of the following is NOT an example of a monosaccharide?

a. Glucose
b. Fructose
c. Sucrose
d. Mannose

245. An exergonic reaction is one that:

a. absorbs energy
b. releases energy
c. involves the addition of water
d. involves the transfer of electrons occurs between reactants

246. What is the difference between an Arrhenius base and a Bronsted-Lowery base?

a. An Arrhenius base accepts protons, and the Bronsted-Lowery base donates hydrogen ions
b. The Arrhenius base releases hydroxide molecules, while the Bronsted-Lowery base donates hydrogen ions
c. The Arrhenius base releases hydroxide ions, and the Bronsted-Lowery base accepts hydrogen ions
d. The Arrhenius base accepts hydrogen ions, and the Bronsted-Lowery base releases hydroxide molecules

247. What are the weak forces that exist between all molecules called?

a. London dispersion forces
b. Dipole-dipole forces
c. Hydrogen forces
d. Chemical bonds

Anatomy and Physiology

248. Which structure in the brain is responsible for arousal and maintenance of consciousness?

a. The midbrain
b. The reticular activating system
c. The diencephalon
d. The limbic system

249. The triceps reflex:

a. forces contraction of the triceps and extension of the arm
b. forces contraction of the biceps, relaxation of the biceps, and arm extension
c. causes the triceps to contract, causing the forearm to supinate and flex
d. causes the triceps to relax and the upper arm to pronate and extend

250. Which cranial nerve is responsible for hearing and balance?

a. CN III
b. CN V
c. CN VIII
d. CN XII

251. Which gland is responsible for the regulation of calcium levels?

a. The parathyroid glands
b. The pituitary gland
c. The adrenal glands
d. The pancreas

252. Which hormone is predominantly produced during the luteal phase of the menstrual cycle?

a. Estrogen
b. Luteinizing hormone
c. Follicle stimulating hormone
d. Progesterone

253. The pancreas secretes what hormone in response to low blood glucose levels?

a. Insulin
b. Glucagon
c. Somatostatin
d. Amylase

254. Which layer of the heart contains striated muscle fibers for contraction of the heart?

a. Pericardium
b. Epicardium
c. Endocardium
d. Myocardium

255. Which part of the cardiac conduction system is the most distal from the initial impulse generation and actually conducts the charge throughout the heart tissue?

a. SA node
b. AV node
c. Purkinje fibers
d. Bundle of His

256. Which blood vessel carries oxygenated blood back to the heart?

a. Pulmonary vein
b. Pulmonary artery
c. Aorta
d. Superior vena cava

257. Which granulocyte is most likely to be elevated during an allergic response?

a. Neutrophil
b. Monocyte
c. Eosinophil
d. Basophil

258. Which vitamin is essential for proper formation of clotting factors?

a. Vitamin A
b. Vitamin K
c. Vitamin B
d. Vitamin C

259. Afferent lymph vessels carry lymph:

a. toward the spleen
b. away from the spleen
c. toward the lymph node
d. away from the lymph node

260. Cricoid cartilage is found on the:

a. alveoli
b. bronchioles
c. bronchi
d. trachea

261. Which of the following is not found in the mediastinum?

a. Xiphoid process
b. Thymus
c. Trachea
d. Vagus nerve

262. What is the proper order of the divisions of the small intestine as food passes through the gastrointestinal tract?

a. Ileum, duodenum, jejunum
b. Duodenum, Ileum, jejunum
c. Duodenum, jejunum, ileum
d. Ileum, jejunum, duodenum

263. The primary function of gastrin is to:

a. inhibit gastric secretion of other hormones
b. stimulate secretion of pancreatic enzymes
c. break down lipids
d. stimulate secretion of gastric enzymes and motility of the stomach

264. The majority of nutrient absorption occurs in the:

a. mouth
b. stomach
c. small intestine
d. large intestine

265. What is the approximate average bladder capacity in an adult?

a. 500 ml
b. 1000 ml
c. 1500 ml
d. 2000 ml

266. Which hormone regulates the amount of urine output?

a. Angiotension I
b. Angiotension II
c. Anti-diuretic hormone
d. Renin

267. Where is the interstitial fluid found?

a. In the blood and lymphatic vessels
b. In the tissues around cells
c. In the cells
d. In the ventricles of the brain

268. Which range represents the normal pH of the body fluids?

a. 7.05 to 7.15
b. 7.15 to 7.25
c. 7.25 to 7.35
d. 7.35 to 7.45

269. What lab values would you expect to see in a patient with respiratory acidosis?

a. Increased $PaCO_2$ and decreased pH
b. Decreased $PaCO_2$ and decreased pH
c. Increased HCO_3^- and decreased pH
d. Decreased HCO_3^- and decreased pH

270. Which testicular cells secrete testosterone?

a. Sertoli cells
b. Leydig's cells
c. Skene's glands
d. Cowper's glands

271. Where does fertilization of an egg by a sperm cell occur?

a. The ovary
b. The uterus
c. The cervix
d. The fallopian tubes

272. Which cells are found in the skin and assist in boosting immune function?

a. Melanocytes
b. Reticular fibers
c. Eccrine glands
d. Langerhans cells

Answer Key and Explanations for Test #2

Reading Comprehension

1. B: The author's primary purpose is to inform the reader about the apparent increase in cases of rickets in developed nations. There is nothing about the essay that suggests persuasion, as the author is simply providing information rather than attempting to persuade the reader to agree with a certain position or opinion. The author provides information but does not necessarily analyze it too closely, so the author's purpose is not to analyze. Additionally, there is little in the essay that indicates a desire to entertain.

2. B: Based on the information at the end of the first paragraph and at the beginning of the second paragraph, the author's main point is that rickets has once again become a problem in some developed nations. (The author starts by noting that this disease is typically seen in nations where children face malnourishment, but that this has not occurred in developed nations for many decades.) Answer choice A suggests a persuasive argument that is not present within the essay. The author does make a final note at the end about rickets becoming a disease of the past, but this is more of a hopeful comment than a call to action. Answer choice C offers information that the author includes as part of the explanation about rickets, but it is supporting information and not the main point. The author singles out the United States and Great Britain but also refers to "other places" where the disease has surprised doctors with its reappearance. This suggests other countries besides the United States and Great Britain, so answer choice D cannot be correct.

3. C: The author clearly mentions the information that is in answer choices A, B, and D. The possibility of a phosphorus deficiency contributing to rickets is noted in the first paragraph. The fact that sunscreen has been identified as a possible vitamin D blocker is mentioned in the third paragraph. The fact that rickets has not been a problem in the United States since the Great Depression is also included in the first paragraph. The author says that *children* in Great Britain are identified as having low vitamin D levels, but there is no mention of vitamin D levels in adults in Great Britain. (This information is actually true, but it is not included in the essay, so answer choice C is correct.)

4. A: If rickets—at least in the United States—was usually a problem that accompanied poor nutrition, and rickets has not been a problem since the Great Depression, the reader can infer that the diet in the United States has improved since the Great Depression. There is nothing in the passage to suggest that people are already taking calcium and vitamin D supplements; in fact, the author notes that doctors are recommending it because people do not have enough calcium and vitamin D. (If they do not have enough, they cannot already be taking the supplements.) The author mentions that sunshine in Great Britain is often in short supply, but there is no discussion of sunshine in the United States. What is more, the author mentions Georgia and North Carolina, neither of which is known for being excessively overcast. And there is no discussion about children's play patterns in the United States, so it cannot be inferred that children in the United States have a vitamin D deficiency because they spend too much time indoors and/or wear too much sunscreen. This discussion is limited to the third paragraph, about Great Britain.

5. D: The author states the exact opposite of the information in answer choice D: far from discouraging breastfeeding, doctors still recommend it. They just encourage nursing mothers to have their vitamin D levels checked and to add a supplement if the levels are low. The author contrasts the developed nations with those that traditionally have poor nutrition and where children suffer from rickets. Developing nations tend to fall into the category of the "third world," so answer choice A is a safe inference. The author includes the information from answer choice B in the final paragraph, so this cannot be correct. Similarly, the author notes in the first sentence of the final paragraph that rickets is not yet considered an epidemic in developed nations but that doctors are concerned about seeing it at all.

6. A: Given the shift in focus from the second paragraph to the third, it is safe to assume that the cause of rickets in Great Britain is linked more to low vitamin D than to low calcium. In fact, the author states outright that doctors in Great Britain believe the cases of rickets are "connected largely to low vitamin D levels." That sunscreen is connected to blocking vitamin D is mentioned, but nothing is said about whether doctors recommend that children wear (or stop wearing) sunscreen. There is no discussion about nursing mothers in Great Britain, so it is impossible to infer anything about the levels of vitamin D in their breast milk. In the first paragraph, low levels of phosphorus are noted as a possible cause of rickets; it is also mentioned that "some researchers" believe this. The word *some* is too vague to determine in any quantity, so it is impossible to say with any certainty if "most researchers" disagree with this.

7. D: In the first paragraph, the author clearly connects rickets with poor nutrition. The author also mentions a time (the Great Depression) when there was poor nutrition in the United States. This would suggest that the term *developed nations* refers to those nations where the citizens have access to adequate nutritional options. There is no mention of a "status quo" anywhere in the passage, so answer choice A makes no sense. Additionally, there is no discussion of politics and economics, so answer choice B cannot be correct. As Great Britain is included among the developed nations but is also noted for having limited sunshine, answer choice C is also incorrect.

8. A: Among the available answer choices, only the word *abundant* makes real sense in the context of the paragraph: Great Britain is not known for having abundant amounts of sunshine. The word *small* makes no sense in the paragraph, since the author is claiming that there is often limited sunshine. The word *expected* does not work, since there is no mention about the amount of sunshine that would be expected. The word *appropriate* does not work, since it is difficult to say whether a certain amount of sunshine is appropriate.

9. A: In the final paragraph, the author simply provides information for preventing and eliminating rickets. Again, this is not a persuasive essay, but the final paragraph is not persuasive in tone. It is largely informative, and the essay would feel incomplete without it. After all, if the essay ended after the third paragraph, the reader would likely wonder about the solution to the problem of rickets. The author says nothing about developing nations in the final paragraph; in fact, the focus is largely on ridding developed nations of a disease that has returned. The author mentions nursing mothers in the final paragraph, but this is in conjunction with the other possible solutions; so, the final paragraph is clearly not focused only on nursing mothers. And answer choice D is too broad for the information in the final paragraph. The author suggests possible options for getting rid of rickets in developed nations, but there is little to infer a "world without rickets" from the information in the paragraph.

10. C: The author focuses on three primary recommendations in the final paragraph: children getting a little sunshine each day (to ensure some vitamin D absorption), people taking vitamin D and calcium supplements, and nursing mothers having their vitamin D levels checked. Limiting television and video games among children is not included as a recommendation, so answer choice C is correct.

11. C: The last sentence of the first paragraph shapes the main idea of the essay: doctors and researchers are concerned about the long-term problems that might result from the chicken pox vaccine. Additionally, the final sentence in the essay notes that there is "ongoing debate about the value of the chicken pox vaccine." These statements offer a clear sense of focus for the essay. The passage does not say that getting the chicken pox vaccine can cause problems with shingles later in life, but this is a supporting point in the passage and not the main idea. Similarly, the author mentions that an increasing number of people in the United States are getting the chicken pox vaccine, but this is a fact the author uses to shape the main point and not the main point itself. The author notes that many children contract chicken pox, but the only mention of adults is in connection with shingles. In fact, there are adults that catch chicken pox, but this is not mentioned in the essay, nor can it be identified as the main point.

12. D: The author's primary purpose is simply to inform the reader about the concerns that many doctors and researchers have about the chicken pox vaccine. The author does not take a clear stand on the issue, and the author does not attempt to persuade the reader either way. The author includes information that analyzes the problem, but the overall focus is on providing information rather than on analyzing. And while the tone of the essay is occasionally playful, the topic is not, so it cannot be said that the author's purpose is to entertain—particularly on so serious a subject.

13. A: The author refers to epidemiologists in conjunction with the potential outbreak of shingles among the people in the United States. This would suggest that an epidemiologist studies diseases among a population. (Looking more closely at the word, the reader can also see a connection to the word *epidemic*, which is the outbreak of disease among a large number of people in a population.) There is no mention of internal organs anywhere in the essay, and as anyone who has had chicken pox knows it reveals itself at the topical level; answer choice B cannot be correct. Chicken pox is indeed a virus (*varicella*), and it is most common among children, but the word *epidemiologist* is not used anywhere near the specific discussion of children and viruses, so answer choice C is too great a stretch. Similarly, the author mentions the outbreak of shingles, but the word *problems* is itself a problem in answer choice D. Shingles is a *disease* that results from a *virus*. What is more, the author makes it clear that shingles is serious enough to go beyond a mere "adult problem," so answer choice D does not have enough support in the passage.

14. A: Nowhere in the passage does the author mention deaths in the United States as a result of chicken pox. The author does, however, note that shingles develops from the same virus as chicken pox. The author states quite clearly that some researchers and doctors believe *not* getting chicken pox might cause problems later on. And the author points out that shingles is a far more serious disease than chicken pox, in part because it attacks elderly adults whose health is already frail.

15. B: The author makes the connection between chicken pox and avoiding shingles: people who contract chicken pox in childhood develop a built-in immunity to shingles later in life. While chicken pox is inconvenient and it might be better to get it over with during childhood, the author says nothing to suggest this as a reason in favor of contracting chicken pox. Answer choice C gets part of the way there, but it does not offer the real reason for contracting chicken pox during childhood: the dormant virus helps *avoid contacting shingles*. And answer choice D is fairly absurd; one should not be in favor of contracting a disease just for the purpose of demonstrating the body's ability to develop a natural immunity to something else.

16. C: The author notes that contracting chicken pox means the individual always has the virus in his or her body. Being around others who have or have had chicken pox creates a kind of booster shot against the disease—just without the actual vaccine. It is a natural immunity boost against the virus, even as it remains in the body. Answer choice A presents a fairly backward way of looking at the issue. What is more, it does not identify the real reason for *being around others who have or have had the disease*, as explained in the correct answer choice, C. Answer choice B provides the desired side effect of catching chicken pox but does not answer the question that is posed. And answer choice D is the preferred result, but again it does not answer the specific question.

17. D: While the author explains that doctors and researchers are concerned about the long-term effects of the vaccine and continue to debate it, there is nothing in the passage to suggest that anyone is advising against it. The author says quite clearly that chicken pox is usually seen as a childhood disease, so it can be inferred that most people contract it during childhood. The author mentions that shingles affects adults over 60, and many of them already have weakened health. This would suggest that their age and state of health increases the problems that shingles brings with it. Finally, the author points out in the first paragraph that vaccines have been invaluable for ridding society of many serious diseases.

18. D: Question 18 requires a little analytical thinking. Avoiding the shingles has two primary parts to it: contracting chicken pox (preferably in childhood) and then being around those who have or have had chicken pox. Extensive vaccinations might not prevent some from catching chicken pox (primarily if they were not vaccinated), but this might mean that people are not around enough people who have had the disease to boost the immunity to it. Answer choice D, therefore, is correct. The author states that the amount of disease in the vaccine is not enough for those who have had chicken pox to boost their immunity to it (among those who have had the vaccine). The author does not, however, mention that the amount in the vaccine is not enough to prevent the shingles later on. Answer choice A cannot be correct. Answer choice B makes little sense. The fears of researchers should not be based on whether there are enough people to use for the study of a disease. Answer choice C has little connection to the question that is posed, so it too cannot be correct.

19. B: The author notes that epidemiologists project the possibility for over 20 million cases of shingles and about 5,000 deaths from the disease. Nothing is mentioned, however, about the time period over which this could occur. One year? Five years? Ten years? Without this information, it is difficult to know how serious of a problem this really is. (In reality, these numbers are projected over the course of fifty years, something that would greatly aid the reader in appreciating the information better.) The names of the researchers would make no difference to the reader's appreciation of the information. The detail about the countries where the vaccine is currently in use has little value for the reader, since these cases/deaths are projected in the United States. The information about the number of people currently vaccinated against chicken pox might be useful elsewhere in the essay, but it does very little to make the author's point stronger in the sentence that is mentioned.

20. C: As noted before, the author does not take a stand but rather focuses on providing information. As a result, the only valid inference from the final statement—when taken in the context of the entire essay—is that the ongoing debate means that researchers continue to evaluate and consider the long term effects of the chicken pox vaccine. Nothing is said about researchers who advise against the vaccine; the only mention is that there is concern and debate. The final sentence notes only "ongoing debate," so there is not enough here (or in the rest of the essay) to infer that researchers believe the vaccine to cause more harm than good. The author says nothing about the number of people who have received or plan to receive the vaccine, so the reader cannot infer that the number of chicken pox vaccinations has decreased.

21. C: An expository composition *exposes* a subject matter by looking at it more closely and analyzing its significance. Additionally, the reader can determine the author's purpose through a process of elimination. As the author takes no clear stand on the issue and does not attempt to convince the reader to assume one side or the other, the passage cannot be persuasive. An investigative piece would require the subject matter to be a mystery that needs to be solved or a problem that needs to be revealed to the public. The author explores the topic and analyzes it more closely, but there is no major reveal within the passage. Finally, an advisory passage would be similar to a persuasive passage in that the author would encourage the reader to take a stand on the issue. As the author does not do that, the only possible answer choice is C.

22. D: The final two sentences of the passage present its main point. The World Health Organization agrees that the remaining samples of the smallpox vaccine should be destroyed, but those within the organization cannot agree about whether all of the samples should be destroyed and when the destruction should occur. Answer choice A cannot be correct because it suggests a persuasive tone that is not within the passage; the author presents information but does not take a stand on the issue. In the same way, answer choice B is incorrect; it offers the polar opposite view that is in answer choice A, but it is still persuasive in tone. And while the author suggests that the United States and Russia cannot agree about whether to destroy the samples, this small part of the passage cannot represent the main point.

23. B: This is something of a trick question that requires careful reading. The author notes that samples of the smallpox virus are still kept in laboratories in Russia. The author also points out that the Soviet Union collapsed in 1991, so it no longer exists. This means that the samples cannot be maintained in a nonexistent political entity. In all reality, the samples are likely to be in the same place in Russia that they were in the Soviet Union (i.e., in the same laboratory). But it is essential to note the relevance of detail in reading comprehension questions, and answer choice B offers a detail that cannot be described as part of the passage.

24. A: The word *consigned* has a range of meanings, depending on the context. It can mean everything from *transferred* to *assign*. In this context, it indicates that the virus has been *sent* to the dustbin of history. What is more, the other answer choices make little sense in the passage. It is illogical to say that the virus has been *refused* to the dustbin of history. Similarly, it cannot be said that the disease is *hidden* in/to the dustbin of history. The sentence indicates that the WHO instituted an inoculation program with the goal of getting rid of the disease among the general population, so it does not make any sense to say that they would want to *keep* it, at least outside of carefully guarded laboratories.

25. A: The last sentence of the second paragraph forges the link between the WHO's ongoing maintenance of the virus samples and the future: the samples provide the means of developing treatment and a vaccine in case of a bioterrorist attack. It makes little sense to argue that the WHO would retain the samples of the virus to prevent the actual attacks of bioterrorism; the relevance seems to be in the need for a response to bioterrorism. While the WHO might very well be interested in continuing research on the virus, there is little in the passage to indicate that this is the reason for retaining the samples. In fact, the author makes a much clearer link between maintaining the samples and responding to bioterrorism. And there is nothing in the passage to suggest that the WHO is prepared to institute a new vaccination program.

26. D: Far from arguing that the WHO is "confident" about the secret samples of the virus, the author makes the parenthetical remark that any unofficial samples were "never confirmed to be real." This does not mean, of course, that they do not exist, but it does suggest that the WHO is not necessarily confident about them. What is more, the author does not focus much on this issue, as the parenthetical remark would indicate. And all other answer choices reflect logical inferences from the passage. The author notes that 70 percent of those who contract smallpox survive; this means that the *majority* of people survive the virus. The author notes at the end of the passage that the WHO cannot agree about whether to destroy all of the remaining samples of the virus. And the author mentions at the beginning of the final paragraph that smallpox is one of the diseases that the WHO believes could be used for acts of bioterrorism.

27. C: In the last paragraph, the author mentions that some researchers—those who support the destruction of the samples—believe that it is no longer necessary to maintain them. This is because a vaccine is already in place to prevent outbreaks of smallpox. Answer choice A does not make much sense because the problem is the potential for outbreaks as a result of bioterrorism. Bioterrorism results not from natural causes of a disease but from deliberate acts of aggression. The disease might be obsolete in the sense of natural outbreaks, but it is not obsolete with regard to the possibility of bioterrorism. Answer choice B cannot be correct because the author makes no connection between the collapse of the Soviet Union in 1991 and the reduced risk of bioterrorism. In fact, the relevance of the researchers' concern suggests that bioterrorism remains a very real threat. Answer choice D goes against the author's statement in the last paragraph that most people are now susceptible to the virus; if they are susceptible, it would stand to reason that few people have been vaccinated.

28. B: Reading between the lines, it is possible to infer two things: there are very few people today who are vaccinated, and among those who were vaccinated during the WHO's inoculation program the effects of the vaccine have worn off. The author notes that the severity of smallpox can create side effects even for those who get the vaccine, but there is no mention about whether people are choosing to be (or not to be) vaccinated. As a result, answer choices A and C cannot be correct. Additionally, the author says little about the public response to smallpox, focusing instead on the concerns of the WHO and other researchers, so answer choice D cannot be correct.

29. D: Even without knowing the meaning of the phrase *at loggerheads*, the reader can deduce from the context that it indicates some kind of clash between the United States and Russia. The sentence states that, "Even the two nations that hold these final samples are at loggerheads about the issue." What is more, this follows the sentences that describe disagreement among scientists about whether to destroy the samples of smallpox virus. As a result, the reader can infer that the expression indicates a dispute of some kind. While the two nations might very well be considering their options, this expression does not offer the sense of disagreement that is implied within the passage. Similarly, the nations might be quietly discussing the issue and might be eager to arrive at a decision, but answer choices B and C do not provide the hint of dispute that is implied in this sentence, as well as the previous sentences.

30. B: The author makes the parenthetical remark that animals do not contract smallpox. At no point in the passage does the author reverse this statement or suggest that animals can contract smallpox, so answer choice B reflects a detail that is not a part of the passage. Answer choice C is incorrect because the author notes that the WHO was instrumental, and successful, in developing a vaccination program to combat smallpox; it also stands to reason that if the program was successful it must have been widespread, affecting many nations around the world. Answer choice B is incorrect because the author mentions in the first paragraph that loss of vision is a potential side effect of smallpox among those who survive. Answer choice D is incorrect because the author states that there were fears of unofficial samples in the hands not just of the Soviet government but of other governments as well.

31. D: The passage starts by providing information on the Black Death and then goes on to discuss the various theories about the cause of the disease. The tone is largely *explanatory*, in that the author explains the information to the reader. A process of elimination can also be useful in this case. There is little about the passage that suggests a *playful* tone. The author does not appear to be overly *concerned* at any point. And the word *definitive* indicates that something is the decisive or ultimate version. The author's tone cannot be described this way, as the author simply informs and explains but does not claim to know everything about the topic.

32. A: There are two parts to the passage, and the main idea should encompass these two parts: the Black Death was devastating for medieval people, and the exact cause or causes of the disease are still under debate. Answer choice B indicates a supporting detail within the second paragraph, but this alone is not enough to present the main point. Answer choice C offers information that is a small detail in the first paragraph; at the same time, answer choice C also goes beyond the information in the passage to suggest a call to action that is not a part of the author's purpose. And like answer choice B, answer choice D only gets half of the information right; it includes details from the first paragraph in the passage but omits the details in the second paragraph.

33. C: At no point does the author mention the Black Death outside of Europe. In fact, the information in answer choice C is correct (or partially correct, since the Black Death was believed to have spread *to* Europe as a result of trading vessels arriving *from* Asia). But it is not a part of the passage. The author does mention, however, that the Black Death reappeared in Europe at various times until the nineteenth century. The author indicates clearly that there remains debate about the cause of the Black Death. And the author states in the first paragraph that medieval doctors did not know what caused the Black Death and thus had no cure for it.

34. B: The author mentions that one theory about the cause of the Black Death notes that there is a similarity between the *spread* of the disease and the Ebola virus. This alone is not enough to suggest that the diseases are related; in fact, the author points out that this is a theory, disputed among scientists and historians, so the fact of a connection between the diseases cannot be inferred. In the last paragraph, the author mentions that the cause(s) of the Black Death remain uncertain. This suggests that there might very well be more than one cause of the disease, and answer choice A can be inferred. In the first paragraph, the author says that between 90 and 95 percent of those who contracted the disease died. This indicates that 5 to 10 percent of those infected survived, so answer choice C can be inferred. In the final sentence of the second paragraph, the author states that the Black Death "permanently changed Europe." Permanent changes have far-reaching effects, so answer choice D can be inferred.

35. A: The author indicates that there are two objections raised to the traditional theory of the bubonic plague: the appearance of the symptoms and the climate of Europe. The explanation about lower lymph nodes is part of the first objection, but this is not the only problem that some have with the flea-and-rat theory. The author mentions that anthrax from cattle has been raised as another alternative theory to the bubonic plague, but the author says nothing about current research seeing a relationship between the diseases. (Again, this is simply one theory among several.) The problem with fleas living long enough to infect so many victims is embedded in the mention of climate, but it too is not the only part of the objection and is thus not enough for a correct answer.

36. C: Question 36 asks the student to identify the author's use of punctuation and what it indicates. Parentheses can solve multiple purposes; in this case, they simply cordon off sentences that are an interesting side note within the discussion but do not fit perfectly into the author's primary flow of thought. The sentences follow from the discussion just before—about how medieval doctors were unsure of the cause—but they create a divergence without the parentheses. Using the parentheses allows the author to include this information while indicating to the reader that it is simply a quick side note. Parentheses seldom create emphasis. In fact, they are used more to minimize the impact of information than to highlight it. And because parentheses do not typically create emphasis, there is no reason to think that the author includes them to strengthen the main point. These brief historical details are more anecdotal than essential, and they do not represent important historical detail. Finally, there is no source noted within the parentheses, so there is no reason to believe that the author is including information from another source here.

37. B: In the first paragraph, the author states that the Black Death "struck and spread quickly," and in the second paragraph, the author points out that some have noticed a similarity between the *spread* of the Ebola virus and the *spread* of the Black Death. This would suggest that the former spreads quickly, just like the latter. While the author points out in the second paragraph that the cause or causes of the Black Death *might* never be known, there is nothing to suggest that it is *impossible* to know the cause or causes. The author says in the first paragraph that there has not been an outbreak of the Black Death since the nineteenth century. This is not enough, however, to assume that modern medicine has ensured another outbreak *will not* occur. The author writes in the first paragraph that medieval people killed cats, believing they were responsible for the Black Death. This suggests a superstitious approach to dealing with the disease. At the same time, the author makes no mention of medieval *doctors* killing cats and does not indicate that the doctors used superstitious approaches to treatment.

38. B: The author's purpose is twofold: to *inform* the reader about the problems that arise with swimmer's ear and to *advise* the reader about how to avoid it. At no point does the author *define* anything, and if there is nothing defined the author cannot *expand* on it. While the author clearly *presents* information, the passage is not *persuasive* in tone; after all, there is nothing to suggest that the author is trying to persuade the reader to believe or do something. Also, while the author does *explain* the details about swimmer's ear, there is little in the passage to indicate that the author is trying to *approve* anything.

39. D: The author says that people who get water in their ear while swimming run the risk of developing swimmer's ear. This is not a guarantee, however. Many people get water in their ear and never develop the condition. Answer choice D cannot be inferred. At the same time, the author says clearly that swimmer's ear results from the bacteria that is in the water making its way into the ear canal. The author notes in the first paragraph that swimmer's ear causes "a bit of swelling" and in the second paragraph that the condition results in the ear canal becoming "inflamed." Taken together, these indicate that swimmer's ear leads to a swelling of the ear canal. Additionally, in the first paragraph, the author notes that the condition is usually seen more as inconvenient than serious, and the author points out in the second paragraph that the problems associated with swimmer's ear can escalate and create more serious side effects.

40. A: Answer choice A is essentially true, but it is not a detail from the passage. Within the passage, the author links swimmer's ear and swimming pools but says nothing about other bodies of water. While the condition might be inferred (however vaguely) to come from other bodies of water, this fact is an implication and not a detail in any of the three paragraphs. The author states in the second paragraph that "otitis externa" is the official name for swimmer's ear. The author notes in the first paragraph that more than two million people in the United States suffer from swimmer's ear annually (and "more than two million" is definitely "over one million"). The author says in the second paragraph that swimmer's ear results from the bacteria in swimming water getting into the ear canal.

41. C: Question 41 asks only for an answer that is *based on the information in the passage*. In all reality, any of the answer choices might technically be true, but the only fact mentioned by the author is that the chlorine in swimming pools is not enough to keep up with all of the bacteria that develops from extra bodies in the water.

42. C: The author says clearly in the third paragraph that the "head-banging" routine (or shaking the head vigorously to release any water in the ear canal) is not advised and offers three options: alcohol to draw the water out, a towel to absorb the water in the ear canal, and a blow dryer.

43. A: Answer choice A is the most complete summary of the information in the passage, which is in two parts: the mysterious sweating sickness broke out in England in the fifteenth and sixteenth centuries, and modern-day scientists have been unable to identify the cause of the disease. The author does say that the doctors in fifteenth and sixteenth century England were mystified by the sweating sickness, but far from suggesting the scientists have begun to understand the disease, the author says clearly that its cause remains a mystery. Additionally, the author mentions that the disease broke out in England in the fifteenth and sixteenth centuries and has not been a problem since, but this is only the content of the first paragraph and ignores the second and third paragraphs entirely; what is more, this summary does not represent the larger point that the author is trying to make about the disease remaining a mystery for scientists. Finally, the author suggests that modern-day scientists have begun to narrow down the options (by presenting the theories about the disease), but there is nothing in the passage to indicate that fifteenth and sixteenth century doctors failed to report on the disease. In fact, in the third paragraph the author mentions doctors of the time who "wrote about the disease," and this clearly indicates that there was reporting on the disease at the time.

44. B: Answer choice B represents a theory about the sweating sickness, that it was caused by a hantavirus. This remains a theory, however, and does not represent a detail from the passage. The other answer choices, on the other hand, do represent details contained in the passage. The author notes in the first paragraph that the sweating sickness struck quickly and often killed victims within a few hours. The author says in the third paragraph that doctors in the fifteenth and sixteenth centuries did not write about seeing any bites from lice or ticks on patients. And the author notes in the first paragraph that the sweating sickness "disappeared from England in the 1570s," which is certainly the latter part of the sixteenth century.

45. D: The author makes several points in the second paragraph: (1) scientists tend to look first to hygiene and sanitation as a cause for epidemics, (2) these tend to be the greatest concern among the poor, (3) the wealthy tend to have better access to good hygiene and sanitation, and (4) the sweating sickness was more likely to strike the wealthy. Taken together, these suggest that the sweating sickness did not result from bad hygiene and sanitation among the poor. As indicated, the author says that the sweating sickness was known for striking the wealthy over the poor. In the final paragraph, the author points out that the sweating sickness is believed to have been spread by human contact. And in the first paragraph, the author states that the deaths from the sweating sickness were not as high as deaths from other epidemics in England (but that the mystery surrounding the disease made it more frightening to people).

46. B: Answer choice B is the only option to contain clearly stated information from the passage. The author says in the third paragraph that hantaviruses are carried by rodents and spread to humans when humans come in contact with the rodents or their waste. The author says nothing about hantaviruses being connected to hygiene and sanitation. The author states clearly in the third paragraph that as far as scientists know hantaviruses cannot be spread from human to human (but only when humans are around rodents or rodent waste). And the author indicates in the third paragraph that the theory of the hantavirus is the "latest theory," but that there are problems with it; these problems make it impossible to say at this time that a hantavirus was the most likely cause.

47. C: The uncertainty of the cause remains a problem for doctors and scientists: if they do not know what caused the sweating sickness, they cannot guarantee that it will not be a problem in the future, and they have no immediate way of preventing it. The author says nothing about modern medical treatments, so answer choice A cannot be correct. The author mentions that doctors in the fifteenth and sixteenth centuries did not notice the bites of lice and ticks on victims of the sweating sickness; there is nothing to suggest that they would not have the observational skills necessary to see these signs. And the author makes no mention of survivors of the disease. This does not mean that people did not survive, nor can it be argued that a low number of deaths indicates a high number of survivals. Instead, this is simply not a part of the passage.

Vocabulary and General Knowledge

48. C: To *bifurcate* is to split into two parts. Within the other answer choices, there is no word with a close enough meaning: to *close* (or shut out), to *glow* (or be illuminated), and to *speak*.

49. C: An *influx* is an arrival in large amounts. For instance, the early twentieth century brought an *influx* of immigrants to the United States through Ellis Island. The word *acceptance* suggests approval, which is not contained in the meaning of *influx* (as there can also be an *influx* of something that is not acceptable). The word *complexity* is related to a degree of complication, and there is nothing in this to connect it to the meaning of *influx*. The word *theory* relates to a proposed idea. Again, there is nothing in this to suggest a clear relationship with *influx*.

50. C: To *substantiate* is to bring evidence to something and thus to *confirm* it. One who *substantiates* a claim confirms its validity. To *inhibit* is to prevent or hold back; this suggests an opposite meaning to *substantiate*. To *assume* is to believe something—with or without *substantiation*. Because *substantiate* indicates the presence of clear supporting evidence, the word *assume* (which suggests the lack of it) cannot be a synonym. To *complete* is to fulfill or accomplish a goal. There is not enough in this meaning to establish a clear relationship with *substantiate*.

51. D: The best definition for the word *typify* is *symbolize*. To *typify* is to indicate a type or *symbol*, to characterize or show an example of. To *obscure* is to make something less clear. Since the act of *typifying* indicates a goal of clarifying, the word *obscure* represents an antonym. To *mock* is to make fun of. There is not enough in the meaning of *typify* to suggest a purpose of *mockery*, so answer choice B cannot be correct. To *announce* is to share important information. There is nothing in this meaning to connect it to the meaning of *typify*.

52. C: The word *sinuous* suggests something that is winding, twisting, or *supple*. The word *ominous* has a negative connotation of impending danger, and while some *sinuous* things can also be *ominous* (such as a *sinuous mountain road that winds up to the very top*), the foundational meaning of the word *sinous* is unrelated to danger. The word *spoiled* suggests overindulgence (in a child) or a state of being rotten (in food). There is nothing in this to connect it to the meaning of *sinuous*. The word *elaborate* suggests a state of complexity. Once again, there is not enough in the meaning of the word *sinuous* to make this connection without a causal relationship.

53. B: The best definition for *transient* is *temporary*. A *transient* ischemic attack is a *temporary* blockage of blood vessels that produces stroke like symptoms without permanent damage. *Intermittent* means stopping and starting, *hesitant* means unsure, and *illusory* means imaginary or fake.

54. D: The word *emaciated* indicates someone or something that is *wasted* from lack of nourishment. The words *vivid* and *fresh* are, to some degree, antonyms, because they indicate a state of being that is healthy and well-nourished. The word *grateful* suggests a positive response to something that is done or given, and this has no immediate relationship with the meaning of *emaciated*.

55. A: Something *irrevocable* cannot be revoked and is thus *binding*. The word *fortunate* indicates that something good has occurred or will occur. While an *irrevocable* decision might also be a *fortunate* one, it might just as easily be (and is often viewed as being) *unfortunate*. The word *unfeasible* means that something is not likely or practical. This has no immediate connection to the meaning of the word *irrevocable*. The word *indefinite* suggests a lack of certainty. This is the opposite of the implied meaning in *irrevocable*, so the words are antonyms instead of synonyms.

56. D: To *abate* is to lessen, decrease, or *reduce*. The opposite of *abate* is *enhance*, since the latter suggests an increase instead of a decrease. To *remove* is to take something away. To *abate* might require that something be taken away, but the meanings are not similar enough, giving the words a conditional relationship. To *revive* is to bring back to life or add to something. Like the word *enhance*, this has a suggestion of increase, making it a possible antonym for *abate*.

57. D: To *extirpate* is to *remove* altogether. The word *assist* suggests help, and there is nothing in here to connect it to the meaning of *extirpate*. The word *define* refers to offering a description or explaining an inherent quality. Again, there is little within this to connect it to the meaning of *extirpate*. The word *provide* indicates an addition or an increase. This makes the word *provide* an antonym for the word *extirpate*.

58. A: Someone who is *feckless* is *incompetent* or ineffective. Someone or something *significant* is of great purpose, so this represents an antonym for *feckless*. Similarly, someone or something *relevant* has immediate purpose and competency, so the word *relevant* is also an antonym. Someone or something that is *headstrong* is stubborn to the point of getting his/hers/its way. Someone *feckless* could also be *headstrong*, but there is not enough in the meanings of these words to suggest an immediate relationship.

59. C: To *constrict* is to *tighten* to an extreme. For instance, the *boa constrictor* squeezes the life out of its prey. The word *collect* indicates an amassing or assembling of items or people. To *collect* is to bring together; to *constrict* is to squeeze forcefully. This has no immediate connection with the meaning of the word *constrict*. To *appreciate* is to show gratefulness for something. Again, there is nothing in this meaning to connect it to the meaning of *constrict*. To *mingle* is to *join*. This has no clear connection to the meaning of the word *constrict*.

60. B: To *goad* is to *force* into action. To *create* is to bring into existence something new. To *bore* is to fail to generate interest for someone or something. To *please* is to make happy. None of these answer choices has any clear relationship with the meaning of the word *goad*.

61. A: The context of the sentence indicates that the school provost chose the proposal that was most *dominantly* favored among the board members. There is nothing in the context of the sentence to suggest that any proposal was deemed *old-fashioned*, so this answer choice cannot be correct. The word *indifferent* makes little sense when applied in place of *prevalent*. (To be *indifferent* is not to care, so it makes no sense for the board members to have an *indifferent favorite* or for the provost to choose a proposal for that reason.) The word *scarce* suggests lack, and since the context of the sentence indicates that the provost chose the proposal that was of interest to most, answer choice D cannot be correct.

62. C: To be *nonchalant* is to be *unconcerned* about an experience, event, or the results of something. The opposite of *nonchalant* is *excited*, so answer choice A cannot be correct. Someone who is *nonchalant* has little emotion about something. Someone who is *cowardly* has strong emotion *not* to do something, so the two words suggest a lack of activity for entirely different reasons. To be *imprudent* is to be unwise about something. A *nonchalant* person might also be *imprudent*, but there is nothing within the meanings of the two words to make an immediate connection.

63. C: To *malinger* is to falsify an illness or *pretend* that is has occurred. To *meet* is to encounter and get to know someone or something. To *prevent* is to hinder something from occurring. To *surge* is to generate a sudden increase. None of these words has any clear connection in meaning with *malinger*.

64. D: Something that is *serrated* has a *jagged* edge. An *unusual* object might also happen to be *serrated*, but a *serrated* edge is not necessarily an *unusual* feature. Someone or something *defiant* is rebellious and ignores or flaunts the rules. There is nothing in this meaning to establish a clear relationship with the meaning of the word *serrated*. Someone or something that is *sad* is in low spirits or is unhappy. The word *serrated* suggests a largely physical quality, while the word *sad* suggests a largely emotional quality. The two words have virtually no similarity in meaning.

65. B: Something *contiguous* is directly next to something else, or is *adjacent*. It is possible for the state of *adjacency* to be *unique*, but this is a largely conditional relationship, and the words have no immediate connection in meaning. Something *indirect* is out of the way or even peripheral. This means that *indirect* functions as a kind of antonym for *contiguous*, which indicates a more immediate relationship between two things. To be *pleased* is to be delighted at the results. There is little within this meaning to connect the words *pleased* and *contiguous*.

66. C: To *obfuscate* is to obscure or *conceal*. To *resemble* is to demonstrate a likeness, so this functions as an antonym for *obfuscate*. To *decide* is to make a choice. There is little in this to suggest an immediate relationship with *obfuscate*. To *surpass* is to exceed or go beyond. Again, there is little clear connection between the word *surpass* and the word *obfuscate*.

67. D: To *portend* is to *forecast* something negative. For instance, in films the ominous music often *portends* frightening events that are about to occur. To *withdraw* is to remove or take away in some form. To *deny* is to claim that something is untrue. To *uncover* is to reveal. None of these answer choices demonstrates any immediate connection to *portend*.

68. C: The context of the sentence indicates that Nina wants to speak privately to her supervisor about his comments but is concerned about *challenging* his authority before the other employees. While discussing the matter with the supervisor at the meeting might very well *disturb* him, the context of the sentence suggests that Nina's motivation stems from her desire not to embarrass her supervisor in public. The sentence clearly states that Nina is *disappointed* by the remarks, so it makes little sense for her to *encourage* her supervisor, either publicly or privately, for the comments that were made. The word *present* makes no sense in the context of the sentence and only confuses the meaning.

69. A: Something that is *immutable* has no mutability or changeability and is thus *unchangeable*. Something that is *breakable* can, by its very nature, be changed, so answer choice A represents a kind of antonym for the word *immutable*. The word *desirable* suggests a state of being wanted, and this has no clear connection to the state of being *unchangeable*. The word *flexible* indicates changeability, so this too is an antonym for *immutable*.

70. B: Something that is *protracted* has been *extended* beyond its expected limits. For instance, a *protracted* legal battle might drag out for years. Something that is *required* is necessary. Something that is *elevated* is raised up, either literally or metaphorically. Neither of these words has any immediate connection to the meaning of *protracted*. Something that is *delayed* is late or has been put on hold. In some contexts, this suggests a possible antonym for the word *protracted*.

71. D: Something that is *viable* has life within it, has options, and has a future. In other words, it is *living*, either literally or figuratively. Something that is *inanimate* has no life within it, so this is an antonym for *viable*. Something that is *reasonable* makes sense or falls within the boundaries of rational explanation. Something that is *likely* is expected to occur. Neither of these words has any direct connection to the meaning of *viable*.

72. C: To be *incessant* is to be *constant* and without ceasing (or cessation). To be *complicated* is to be difficult or convoluted. To be *uncertain* is to be without certainty and lacking definition. To be *frightening* is to be scary or alarming. None of these words has a meaning with any connection to the meaning of *incessant*.

73. C: Something that is *negligible* has little value, is insignificant, or is *minor*. The word *adequate* suggests an acceptable or approved amount; this could function as a possible antonym for *negligible*. Similarly, the word *significant* means the very opposite of the word *negligible*, so it is an antonym. The word *careless* suggests someone who *neglects* to pay attention to responsibility, but the word *neglect* and the word *negligible*, while related in origin, have entirely different meanings.

74. A: To *accost* is to *confront* or challenge someone. A person who *accosts* someone else might very well *insult* or *mock* the other person at the same time, but the verb *accost* does not have the immediate implication of a negative confrontation. In some cases, to *accost* is to issue a justifiable demand. To *evade* is to avoid, and this is the very opposite meaning of *accost*.

75. C: To *retreat* is to back off or *withdraw*. For instance, an army that *retreats* pulls its soldiers back from battle. To *provide* is to offer or give necessary or useful items. To *anger* is to cause wrath in someone else. There is no clear relationship between the meanings of either of these words and the meaning of *retreat*. To *contain* is to hold on to something or *enclose* it. The word *retreat* has the implication of getting out or getting away, so the word *contain* represents a kind of antonym for *retreat*.

76. D: A *dichotomy* is a *split* between two items or ideas. In politics, there is often a clear *dichotomy* between those on the right and those on the left. The word *formation* suggests the start of something. There is nothing in the meaning of this word to indicate a connection to the meaning of *dichotomy*. The word *decision* indicates a clear choice; while someone might make a *decision* about which side of a *dichotomy* to support, these words have a causal relationship rather than a synonymous one. The word *interruption* indicates a pause, even a *split* in time. But this stretches the possibility of a synonym for *dichotomy*. A *dichotomy* is a true split, as if with a cleaver (whether literal or metaphorical). There is the implication of a chasm between the two sides. An *interruption* is simply a pause that may or may not be filled with something else. For instance, one person who *interrupts* another often does so by jumping in and adding something of his or her own.

77. B: To be *solicitous* is to be *attentive*, often to the point of the attention being unpleasant, although there is not necessarily a purely negative quality in the word; a nurse who is *solicitous* is carefully *attentive* to his or her patients. The word *plentiful* suggests excess, and while a *solicitous* person can be described as *plentiful* in attention, the word *plentiful* is not always related directly to attention. Someone who is *ignorant* has limited knowledge and is thus not paying attention at all. This functions as a kind of antonym for *solicitous*. Someone who is *stubborn* refuses to go along with what is asked or required. There is no clear relationship between the word *stubborn* and the word *solicitous*.

78. A: A *trajectory* is a proposed *direction* that someone or something can take. A college graduate's future career can have an expected *trajectory* (where the graduate intends to go and how he or she intends to proceed in the career). A missile can have an expected *trajectory* (striking what it is supposed to strike). The word *excitement* relates to eager anticipation over some expected event. While both *excitement* and *trajectory* have an implied suggestion of anticipation, there is little else to connect the meanings of the words. The word *simplification* means a reduction down to the bare basics. There is nothing in this to suggest a clear relationship with the word *trajectory*. And while determining a *trajectory* requires a certain amount of *calculation*, the connection between these words is largely causal.

79. D: Something that is *unwarranted* is unnecessary or even *inappropriate*. Clearly, Agnes's comment is not acceptable, so the teacher calls her out for it. If the comment is *inappropriate*, it is certainly not *justifiable*, so the latter word is an antonym for *unwarranted*. Agnes's comment might be rooted in a measure of *bias*, making it *inappropriate*, but this suggests a cause-and-effect relationship instead of a synonymous one. If Agnes's remark is *unwarranted*, it is definitely not *essential*, so answer choice C cannot be a synonym.

80. A: To be *intemperate* is to lack any sense of personal restraint and thus to be *unrestrained*. For example, the Temperance Movement in the United States began in an effort to help people restrain themselves against overconsumption of alcoholic beverages (and ultimately evolved into a no-alcohol policy). Someone who is *unconcerned* is largely indifferent to what is happening. This has no clear connection with the meaning of *intemperate*. Someone who is *idle* is doing nothing and wasting time. While this meaning is not directly opposite the meaning of *intemperate*, the word *intemperate* does suggest some form of excess action—and the word *idle* suggests no action at all. To be *organized* is to be prepared, have everything planned, and even have a sense of control. This suggests a type of antonym for *intemperate*, since one who is *unrestrained* is certainly not *organized*.

81. C: Something that is *onerous* represents a great burden and is, as a result, very *demanding*. Something *trivial* is small and unimportant, making this word a kind of antonym for *onerous*. Something *motivating* encourages action; it might require *motivation* to complete an *onerous* task, but the relationship between these words is essentially causal rather than synonymous. Something that is *urgent* requires immediate attention. Again, it might be possible for something *onerous* to be *urgent* as well, but this indicates a cause-and-effect relationship instead of a direct similarity in meanings.

82. A: *Heterogeneous* indicates a measure of *difference*, things that are unique or distinct. (This is contrasted with *homogeneous*, which suggests direct similarity.) Something *heterogeneous* might also be *unusual*, but there is nothing *unusual* in the fact of *heterogeneity*. The word *clear* indicates something obvious or easy to understand. There is nothing in this meaning to suggest a similarity to the meaning of the word *heterogeneous*. The word *comparable* indicates a measure of sameness; this functions as an *antonym* for *heterogeneous*.

83. A: To be *overwrought* is to be pushed to an extreme, to be very *agitated*. To be *respected* is to bear the appreciation of peers and others. There is little in the meaning of this word to suggest a relationship with the word *overwrought*. To be *indifferent* is to lack interest or not to care about something; someone who is *overwrought* cares very much about what is happening, so the word *indifferent* represents an opposite for the word *overwrought*. One who is *overwrought* is *excessive* in emotion and concern. At the same time, it is possible to see *excess* in many other areas, so the word *excessive* describes the word *overwrought*. The two words are not, however, synonyms.

84. B: Someone who is in his or her *dotage* is in a state of *senility*. *Senility* suggests a certain weakness, so the word *strength* is a kind of antonym for the word *dotage*. The word *balance* also indicates a measure of well-being, so there is a hint of an opposite in this word as well. The word *position* indicates a role that is played; there is no immediate relationship between the word *position* and the word *dotage*.

85. D: The word *puerile* has its roots in the Latin word for *child*. As it has evolved in English usage, the word *puerile* now suggests someone who is *childish* in behavior, with a negative denotation of immaturity. The word *youthful* has a positive connotation of being young, healthy, even *childlike*—to the same thing as *childish*—so it is not a strong synonym for *puerile*. To be *sophisticated* is to have a measure of maturity; this functions as a kind of antonym for *puerile*. To be *virtuous* is to be morally upright; there is little in this meaning to connect the words *virtuous* and *puerile*.

86. C: Something that is *putative* is assumed or *accepted*, with or without solid evidence. Something or someone that is *chosen* has the mark of preference; there is little in this to connect the meaning of the word *chosen* with the meaning of the word *putative*. Something *factual* has solid support and evidence. Since *putative* indicates *acceptance*, with or without *fact*, the words are closer to being antonyms than synonyms. To be *effective* is to be useful in some form. There is no immediate relationship between this word and the word *putative*.

87. D: To *enumerate*, from the Latin "to number" or "to count," suggests a measure of clear *specification*. A patient might ask a doctor to *enumerate* the steps that he or she should take for better health. This is a request for *specific* details, not vague ideas. To *refuse* is to reject in some form. To *plead* is to beg. To *include* is to bring someone or something in. None of these words has any direct relationship in meaning to the meaning of the word *enumerate*.

88. B: Something that is *intangible* is unclear, lacking in substance, or *vague*. Something that is *sudden* is unexpected; it is possible for something to be *intangible* and *sudden*, but the relationship between the words is causal rather than synonymous. Something that is *forthright* is straightforward; this can function as a possible antonym for *intangible*. Similarly, something that is *definite* is clear; this is a strong antonym for *intangible*.

89. D: A *relapse* is a decline, a reversion of the good, or a *setback*. *Prevention* is useful to avoid a *setback*, but this relationship is more one of cause and effect (or even chronology). An *endearment* is a presentation of fondness, so there is no clear relationship between this word and the word *relapse*. A *progression* is a moving forward; this is the opposite of *relapse*, so the words are antonyms.

90. C: Something that is *definitive* is clear and precise; it can also suggest an *ultimate* quality. Something *absurd* is ridiculous. It is possible for an *absurdity* to be *definitive*, but the relationship between these words suggests cause and effect. Something that is *definitive* suggests a measure of completion, so the word *incomplete* is a kind of antonym. It is possible to *prefer* something *definitive*, but the quality of being *definitive* does not guarantee *preference*.

91. B: To *conflate* is to *merge* in some form. There is nothing about the inherent meaning of *conflation* that suggests *falsification*, so the two words are unrelated, either as antonyms or as synonyms. To *anticipate* is to expect something. Again there is nothing in this meaning to suggest a connection to the meaning of the word *conflate*. To *conflate* is to bring together; this bringing together might or might not suggest *expansion*, but *expansion* does not always come about through *conflation*.

92. D: A *congenital* condition is *innate* or in existence from birth. A *contracted* condition is one that is caught rather than inherent, so these words are antonyms. A *congenital* condition is likely to be a *lifelong* one, but the meaning of *lifelong* does not equate directly to *innateness*. For instance, someone can *contract* an illness that causes *lifelong* problems. Something *additional* is in excess. A *congenital* quality is *innate* for the one who experiences it, so it cannot be said to be *additional*.

93. A: To *gestate* is to *conceive* or begin in some form. To *provide* is to give or offer something. To *delete* is to remove something. To *remind* is to bring back to memory something that has (potentially) been forgotten. None of these words have any direct connection in meaning to the meaning of *gestate*.

94. D: Something that is *mordant* is biting in tone or *disrespectful*; to issue *mordant* criticism is to criticize in an offensive way. Something *elegant* is *sophisticated* or *graceful*—not necessarily an antonym for the word *mordant*, but it is unlikely that the qualities of *mordancy* and *elegance* would coexist. Something that is *soothing* is kind or gentle; this is a kind of antonym for the word *mordant*. Something that is *joking* is playful and not serious; to be *joking* can also be biting or *disrespectful*, but it does not necessarily have to be. The words cannot be synonyms.

95. C: To *transmute* is to *change* in some way. To *annoy* is to irritate; to *maintain* is to preserve or continue; to *charge* is to burden, allege, or establish a price on something. None of these words offers a clear connection in meaning to the word *transmute*.

96. B: To *circumscribe* is to go around and hold in, to confine, and to *enclose*. To *continue* is to keep going in some way. To *converse* is to engage in conversation. These words are unrelated in meaning to the word *circumscribe*. To *permit* is to allow; because *circumscription* suggests prevention or hindrance, the word *permit* is an antonym for the word *circumscribe*.

97. C: The word *prehensile*, with a Latin root meaning "to grasp," indicates *greed*. A *gentle* person is kind and gracious. While the words are not antonyms, it is not likely that a *gentle* person would also be *prehensile*. A *clever* person is intelligent and quick-witted. There is nothing in this meaning to suggest a connection to the meaning of *prehensile*. A *gracious* person is generous, so the words *gracious* and *prehensile* are antonyms.

Grammar

98. B: To *imply* is to give a suggestion; to *infer* is to receive that suggestion. In this sentence, Detective Melchior tries to *imply* something to his sidekick, but the sidekick cannot *infer* the meaning (i.e., the sidekick does not understand the suggestion). Answer choice B places the words in the correct order: *imply, infer*.

99. C: A sentence that is in the active tense has the subject *doing* the action instead of *receiving* it. The opposite of active tense is passive tense: the subject is receiving the action or *being acted upon*. In answer choice C, the fashion designer is *presenting* the collection—that is, he is doing the action of presenting. In answer choice A, the child is receiving the gifts from friends (*was given presents by his friends*). In answer choice B, the marathon winner is receiving the medal from the awards committee (*was rewarded...by the awards committee*). In answer choice D, the duck a l'orange is in the process of being eaten—that is, the duck is being acted upon (*was quickly devoured by the eager culinary students*).

100. C: The word *much* suggests an uncountable amount, while the word *many* suggests something countable. *Time* is uncountable, so the speaker of the sentence requires the form *much*. The speaker's *tasks* are certainly countable, so he or she requires the form *many*. Answer choice C places the words in the correct order: *much, many*.

101. D: Question 4 presents a similar situation as question 3, although now it is a choice between *less* (which is uncountable) and *fewer* (which is countable). Edwina had *less* time than she anticipated, so she went to the lane that said "Ten Items or *Fewer*." Despite the signs that read *Ten Items or Less* in grocery stores across the United States, this form is actually incorrect. If the shopper can count the number of items in his or her cart, he or she will know if there are ten items or *fewer*.

102. B: Capitalization rules require that the main words that describe the official name of a conflict be capitalized. In other words, the correct form is *World War I*, with all parts capitalized. The other answer choices, with the mix of capitalized words, cannot be correct.

103. C: Capitalization rules state that prepositions do not need to be capitalized in formal names, unless those prepositions are longer than four letters. In the case of question 6, the correct form then would be *Siege of Leningrad*, with the words *Siege* and *Leningrad* capitalized. The short preposition *of* does not need to be capitalized.

104. A: The words *earth*, *sun*, and *moon* are not capitalized unless they are listed with other planets. In this sentence, the inclusion of *Saturn*, *Neptune*, and *Jupiter* requires that *Earth* and *the Sun* be capitalized (even if the word *the* is added before *Sun*). In this case, the word *the* is not necessary before *Earth* because *Earth* is being referred to among the formal names of planets. (*The Sun* is always referred to with the article.)

105. D: Question 8 asks for the correct abbreviation for *milligrams*, which is *mg*. So the doctor prescribes *4 mg* of the medication to be taken daily. Answer choices A and B are meaningless. Answer choice C prescribes *4 meters* to the patient—clearly, not what the doctor has ordered.

106. A: The phrase *Janet and* _______ is an appositive form that expands *My two friends*. Because *My two friends* is the subject of the sentence, the pronoun in the appositive phrase should be the subjective case: *she*. The form *her* is in the objective case, as is the form *them*. The form *they* is in the subjective case, but the context of the sentence calls for *two friends*, and *Janet and they* would make for more than two.

107. C: The pronoun *Somebody* is singular, so it requires a singular verb: *has*. (*Somebody has been in my house!*) The verb *have* is plural. The verbs *will* and *might* make no sense when connected directly to *been*. In both cases, the verbs need the form *have* to follow immediately before *been*. (That is, *will have been* or *might have been*.)

108. C: The context of the sentence shows that the blank follows a preposition, making the expression the object of the preposition. Pronouns that function as the object of the preposition should be in the objective case: *us students*. (To check for sure, simply remove the word *students* since it acts as a kind of appositive and is not essential to the meaning of the sentence: *the financial burden placed on us*.) The form *we* is subjective in case. The form *those* makes no sense, as the speaker is the head of the student council and thus also a student. The form *them students* is never correct.

109. A: The rules of hyphenation require a hyphen after the first word to indicate that it should be attached to another word: *part- and full-time*, because this would otherwise be *part-time and full-time*. The hyphens are required to indicate that the combination of the two words represents a single adjective. The slashes are never used to create adjectives.

110. C: The word *take* suggests direction away from someone, and the word *bring* suggests direction toward someone. In other words, the speaker wants the person hearing him or her to *take* the tea away and to *bring* something else. Answer choice C offers the correct order of these words: *take, bring*.

111. A: The verb *ought* can work on its own, without a helping verb (such as *had* or *should*). In fact, *should* and *ought* are similar in meaning, so the expression *should ought* is largely redundant. The word *had* on its own makes little sense in the sentence.

112. C: Because the name *Sherlock Holmes* is singular, the possessive form requires an apostrophe and the letter *s* to follow: *Sherlock Holmes's*. The apostrophe alone is only correct for a word that is already plural. The apostrophe before the final *s* alters the name of *Sherlock Holmes* to *Sherlock Holme*. The lack of any apostrophe fails to recognize the context of the sentence, which calls for the possessive case.

113. B: The context of the sentence indicates a single novel that has a surprising solution for Linus. As a result, the singular possessive *mystery's* must be correct. The form *mysteries* is plural but has no possession. The form *mysteries'* is plural possessive, which the context of the sentence contradicts (in the singular *detective novel*). The form *mysterie's* is never correct.

114. D: The sentence has a plural subject—*Both Hugo and Camille*—so it requires a plural verb, *are*. The forms *is* and *was* are singular. The form *were* is plural, but the past tense of *were* contradicts the present tense indicated by *participate* later in the sentence. If Hugo and Camille *were* members of the local rotary club but no longer are, they would probably not still be participating in the annual auction.

115. A: The form *rise* is intransitive (requiring no object), while the form *raise* is transitive (requiring a noun/pronoun object). For example, we *rise* from bed every morning, but we *raise* a flag. The coach calls upon the team to *rise* to the challenge (no object) and *raise* the bar (the word *bar* representing an object) in this context. All other answer choices are incorrect for including the wrong words or order of the words.

116. D: The form *lie* is intransitive, and the form *lay* is transitive. The speaker says that the listener should not *lie* down (no object) but wait until he/she can *lay* new sheets (object: sheets). All other answer choices are incorrect for including the wrong words or order of the words.

117. A: The form *their* is a possessive pronoun; the form *they're* is a contraction for *they are*; the form *there* indicates direction or location. Answer choice A is correct because it correctly orders the words to identify *their car* (possessive pronoun identifying the owner of the car), identify that *they're [they are] going to Evan's house*, and noting that they will stay *there* (at Evan's house) until the car is repaired. All other answer choices are incorrect for including the wrong words or order of the words.

118. C: The form *between* should be used for two people, while the form *among* should be used for more than two people. Answer choice C is correct because it accurately fills the sentence in with *Between the two of us* and *among all ten of the board members*. All other answer choices are incorrect for including the wrong words or order of the words.

119. C: A colon should be used to introduce a list of items, only when the expression "the following" (or "as follows") appears before the list. Answer choice A does not include any punctuation between the introduction to the list and the list itself. Answer choice B uses a semicolon, thus creating a fragment in the second part of the sentence. Answer choice D uses a comma, which is not correct to introduce a list.

120. D: A semicolon may be used between items in a list when those items contain internal commas. In the case of cities and states, it is customary to use a semicolon between each city/state listing. Answer choice A fails to use any commas or semicolons, which creates confusion in separating the items in the list. Answer choice B uses only commas, which similarly creates confusion in separating each city/state listing. Answer choice C fails to use commas to separate the city from its respective state, which is incorrect.

121. D: Answer choice D correctly offsets the name *Mateo* with commas, thereby indicating direct address. Answer choice A only uses a comma before *Mateo*, and a comma is necessary after the name as well. Answer choice B fails to add a comma before *Mateo* but adds a semicolon after it. This only creates a fragment. Answer choice C uses a colon, but the context of the sentence does not require a colon. (Colons can be used to introduce defining qualities or characteristics. In this case, nothing is defined. The rest of the comment is simply completed after the speaker addresses Mateo by name.)

122. B: The form *beside* suggests adjacency, as in one person is standing *beside* another. The form *besides* suggests exclusion, as in everyone *besides* Anne was invited to the party. In the sentence, the form *besides* belongs in the first blank because only Marine and Elsa want to go to the pool. The form *beside* belongs in the second blank because Marine and Elsa plan to get some sun *beside* the pool.

123. D: The comma correctly separates the two parts of the sentence with a slight pause. Having no internal punctuation is wrong, since there needs to be some sort of separation between the two phrases. As the sentence contains a single independent clause instead of two independent clauses, the semicolon only succeeds in creating two fragments. Colons are useful for introducing defining statements, but in this case the colon makes little sense, as the second part of the sentence simply completes the initial statement. (For instance, saying the first part of the sentence without the second makes very little sense.)

124. B: The sentence is interrogative, so it requires a question mark at the end. The speaker is asking Jeannette when the guests will arrive. The statement is complete in itself, and there is no sense that the speaker trails off; as a result, the ellipsis cannot be correct. The statement is a question and not a declaration, so the period at the end cannot be correct. The speaker is not commanding Jeannette or making an exclamatory statement, so the exclamation point is incorrect.

125. C: The pronoun phrase *Either...or* is singular, so the statement *Either Eleanor or Patrick* requires a singular verb. The verb *should* makes no sense in the sentence, at least without the addition of *be*. The verbs *are* and *were* are both plural.

126. D: The context of the sentence indicates that Edgar was unable to attend the function, due to the trains. As a result, the verb *would have liked*, with its hint of the past-tense conditional, fits best. The event occurred; Edgar could not attend; he *would have liked* to attend, however. The verb *had liked* does not fit the context of Edgar's being unable to attend. The verb *would like* has a future connotation that does not work in the past tense context of the sentence (with the event having occurred). The verb *was liking* has a quality of the present tense ongoing, and this does not fit the indication of the event having passed.

127. A: The verb *were* is correct because the sentence it subjunctive in tone; subjunctive statements indicate something that could be, should be, would be, but are not. In this sentence, the context suggests that the speaker should be more diligent but is not. The verb *are* does not work in the sentence in any context. The verb *am* does not fit the conditional tone that is suggested by the use of *would* in the main clause. The verb *was* is not correct in a subjunctive sentence.

128. B: This sentence is also subjunctive, as the subjunctive tense can also indicate a demand or requirement. When that occurs, the correct usage is the *to be* version of a verb, but without the *to*. In other words, *She insisted that the children be in the house no later than four o'clock*. The verb *will be* almost works, but the use of the strict future form *will* does not work with the conditional tone of the sentence. (The form *would* is more correct.) The verb *are* sounds awkward in the reading of the sentence. Again, the conditional tone requires a more conditional sounding verb, and *are* is a strict present tense verb. The tone of the sentence suggests an event in the future, so the past tense verb *were* makes little sense here.

129. D: The context of the sentence calls for the phrase *to be cleaned*, indicating a future activity: *The car needs to be cleaned before we leave for our trip*. The form *cleaned* is an incorrect colloquial usage with a past tense context. The car is certainly not going to clean itself, so the infinitive *to clean* makes no sense in the sentence. The form *cleaning* works no better than *cleaned*, although it would fit as a gerund if it had the article *a* before it: *The car needs a cleaning.*

130. A: The word in the blank is an adverb that modifies the verb *went* and answers the question *How [did he go forward]?* As a result, the correct answer is the adverb form *cautiously*. The word *caution* is a noun, and nouns cannot modify verbs. The word *cautious* is an adjective, and adjectives can only modify nouns and pronouns. The form *cautioned* is either a past tense verb or an adjective, neither of which makes sense in the context of the sentence.

131. C: The form *well* is an adverb that is always used to indicate health. In other words, *she felt well*; she cannot feel *good* when describing health. (The form *good*, however, can be used to describe how someone feels about an action or decision, i.e., *She felt good about her decision to attend the state university.*) The forms *better* and *best* are both adjectives; additionally, neither makes sense next to the word *enough*.

132. C: While the word *important* could work in some circumstances, this sentence has a clear clue to indicate the need for a word before it: the presence of the article *a*, which cannot go before a word that begins with a vowel. (Some sentences will include the option for a(n) to indicate either possibility. As that is not the case here, the student can assume that the first word in the blank must start with a consonant.) Among the answer choices, the only one that makes sense and is grammatically correct is the adverb-adjective form *really important*, with the adverb *really* modifying the adjective *important*. The expression *more important* could work, except that the use of *more* indicates a qualifier; as the sentence does not indicate what the event is *more important than*, it fits the sentence awkwardly.

133. D: The adverb form *barely* should usually modify an adjective or another adverb. In other words, the sentence suggests that Cedric *had barely any food*—indicating that *barely* modifies the adjective *any* and indicates the limited amount of food that Cedric had. The form *barely had any* modifies the verb *had*, which is fairly awkward. After all, how does one *barely have* something? (One either *has* something, or one does not.) The expression *had any* makes no sense in the sentence, especially as the context indicates that Cedric had very little (if any) food. The expression *had barely no* is never correct because both *barely* and *no* are negatives. The combination creates the dreaded double negative.

134. B: The form *prettier* should be used to compare two entities; the form *prettiest* should be used to compare three or more entities. In the first blank, Meg is one entity, while Beth and Jo are combined into a single entity for the comparison. As a result, the form *prettier* is correct here. The second blank is a comparison of all four girls individually, so Amy can be said to be the *prettiest* of them. The correct order of the words is *prettier, prettiest.*

135. B: The word *unique* cannot be qualified. Something is either *unique*, or it is not. Something cannot be *more or less unique*, as the state of uniqueness would no longer exist. This means that the only correct form can be the word *unique* by itself. The forms *a most unique* and *a more unique* both qualify the word. The form *uniquest* is not even a word.

136. D: The form *further* should be used to describe metaphorical distance; the form *farther* should be used to describe literal distance. Therefore, *He refused to consider further*[metaphorical distance] *which route to the store would be best so he would not have to go farther* [literal distance] *than necessary*. The mention of the *store* clarifies that the unnamed *he* is making a physical journey, so the correct order of the words is *further, farther.*

137. C: As with *good* and *well*, the forms *bad* (adjective) and *badly* have distinct uses when describing health versus personal feelings. In other words, the form *bad* should describe personal feelings (just as the form *good* does), while the form *badly* should describe health. And because the form *badly* is an adverb, it can be used to describe someone's activity or performance. The first blank in the sentence describes Zenaida's personal feelings: *She felt bad* (about how the child was doing). The second blank describes the child's performance: *the child was doing so badly in the math class*. The correct order of the words should be *bad, badly.*

138. A: The word *council* describes a body of people who make decisions. The word *counsel* describes the advice that is given. As a result, Jerome submitted his issue to the *council* (or a group of people) in hopes of receiving *counsel* (or advice) from them. The correct order of the words is *council, counsel.*

139. A: The word *advise* is a verb that describes the act of providing guidance. The word *advice* is the noun that describes the actual guidance that is given. This means that the speaker of the sentence is asking that someone *advise* him/her (or provide guidance) because he/she needs some helpful *advice* (actual guidance) to make a decision about a contractor. The correct order of the words is *advise, advice.*

140. D: To *elude* is to get away from in some way. (The suspect was able to *elude* the police.) To *allude* is to make a reference of some kind. (Writers often *allude* to the work of other writers.) In the sentence, the first blank suggests that true emotions *elude* (or get away from) people. The second blank indicates that a poet was trying to *allude* to (or refer to) this in his/her work. The correct order of the words is *elude, allude.*

141. B: The correct plural form of *bus*, when it refers to the vehicle that carries people, is *buses*. The form *busses* is based on the verb *buss*, which means *to kiss*. The singular form *bus* cannot be correct because the sentence clearly indicates that Carl took more than one bus. The form *bus's* is singular possessive, and this makes no sense in the context of the sentence.

142. B: The context of the sentence suggests that the material following the colon is the actual quote from the professor. This means that it belongs in quotation marks. Titles of poems are punctuated according to the poem's length: a shorter poem's title goes in quotation marks, while a longer poem's title is italicized. Either punctuation would be acceptable here, but not both together, as in choice C. If quotes were used here, they would need to be single quotes, since the poem is referenced within a larger quoted text. Choice D places the close quotation mark inside the period, which is always wrong.

143. D: The correct spelling is *victorious*. All other words in the sentence are spelled correctly.

144. D: The correct spelling is *occurrence*. All other words in the sentence are spelled correctly.

145. A: The word that is required in the blank is a transition word that indicates a reversal or contrast, since the first half of the sentence indicates a negative situation, while the second half indicates a successful resolution. Of the choices listed, the only option that provides a contrasting transition is *however*.

146. A: The sentence in answer choice A is a complete, grammatically-correct sentence. The sentences in answer choices B and C both contain verb tense errors, and the sentence in answer choice D is a run-on sentence.

147. B: The sentence in answer choice B is grammatically correct and the verb tense is logically consistent throughout. The sentence in answer choice A pairs *it* with the plural verb *are*. The sentence in answer choice C uses the participle *getting* in place of the past tense verb *got*. Finally, the sentence in answer choice D switches from past tense to present tense (and the wrong form of present tense at that).

Mathematics

148. B: A percentage is a number of hundredths; in this case $75\% = \frac{75}{100}$. To find a percentage of a number you multiply the number by the percentage in fraction or decimal form. So 75% of 500 = $500 \times \frac{75}{100} = \frac{37500}{100} = 375$.

There is an alternative way to solve this problem. 75% is a common enough percentage that it's worth committing to memory its equivalent fraction: 75% is $\frac{3}{4}$ (which $\frac{75}{100}$ reduces to). So we're really looking for $\frac{3}{4}$ of 500. One quarter of 500 is $500 \div 4 = 125$, so three quarters of 500 is $125 \times 3 = 375$.

149. A: When performing a series of operations, we always perform the operations in parentheses first. We also always perform multiplications and divisions before additions and subtractions, so in this case even without the parentheses the order of operations would be the same. In any case, we first carry out the multiplications in the parentheses: $(7 \times 5) + (8 \times 2) = 35 + 16$. Now we carry out the addition: $35 + 16 = 51$.

150. D: When performing a series of operations, we always perform the operations in parentheses first. So we'll start with the divisions in parentheses: $(8 \div 2) \times (12 \div 3) = 4 \times 4$. Now we carry out the multiplication: $4 \times 4 = 16$. In this case, the parentheses didn't really matter; if we had just carried out the operations left to right we would have obtained the same answer. But that isn't always true: for instance, $(12 \div 2) \times 3 = 6 \times 3 = 18$, but $12 \div (2 \times 3) = 12 \div 6 = 2$.

151. D: A number is a **factor** of another number if the first number can be multiplied by some integer to get the second number. Equivalently, a number is a factor of another number if a division of the second number by the first number does not leave a remainder (or in other words leaves a remainder of zero). In this case, there is no integer we can multiply by 5 to get 36, and dividing 36 by 5 leaves a remainder of one. Either of these facts tells us that 5 is not a factor of 36. Neither 7 nor 8 can be multiplied by another number to get 36; dividing 36 by 7 leaves a remainder of 1, and dividing 36 by 8 leaves a remainder of 4. So 7 and 8 aren't factors of 36 either. However, we *can* multiply 9 by another number to get 36: $9 \times 4 = 36$. And so dividing 36 by 9 does not leave a remainder. So 9 is a factor of 36.

152. C: We can, of course, easily solve this problem by typing the operation into a calculator. But we can do it without a calculator as well. We write the numbers one above the other, and then start by multiplying 75 by 4: $5 \times 4 = 20$, write down the 0 and carry the 2, $7 \times 4 = 28$, plus 2 = 30:

$$\begin{array}{r} \overset{2}{7}5 \\ \times 34 \\ \hline 300 \end{array}$$

Now we multiply 75 by 3, writing this result one space to the left: $5 \times 3 = 15$, write down the 5 and carry the 1, $7 \times 3 = 21$, plus 1 = 22:

$$\begin{array}{r} \overset{1}{7}5 \\ \times 34 \\ \hline 300 \\ 225 \end{array}$$

Finally, we add the two lines together:

$$\begin{array}{r} 75 \\ \times 34 \\ \hline 300 \\ 225 \\ \hline 2550 \end{array}$$

153. B: To solve for a variable in an algebraic equation, we can isolate the variable on one side by reversing any operations done to it, carrying out the reverse operation on both sides. In this case, 372 is added to x; the reverse operation is *subtracting* 372: we can get rid of the 372 on the left side of the equation by subtracting 372 from both sides:

$$x + 372 = 853$$
$$x + 372 - 372 = 853 - 372$$
$$x = 481$$

154. A: 0.25 is a decimal that comes up often enough it's worth committing to memory, so you may know the answer to this without having to work anything out. Even if you don't, however, it's still possible to solve for it. The second space after the decimal is the hundredths space, so 0.25, with two digits after the decimal point, is equal to $\frac{25}{100}$. This can be simplified: $\frac{25 \div 25}{100 \div 25} = \frac{1}{4}$.

155. B: To convert a decimal into a fraction, we first note the place value of the rightmost digit in the decimal. In this case, 0.85 has two digits after the decimal point, and the space of the second digit after the decimal point is the hundredths space. Now, we take the digits after the decimal, and make them the numerator of a fraction with that denominator: in this case that gives us $\frac{85}{100}$. Finally, we simplify if possible. In this case, both the numerator and denominator are divisible by 5, so we can write $\frac{85}{100} = \frac{85 \div 5}{100 \div 5} = \frac{17}{20}$.

156. B: Perhaps the quickest way to solve this problem is to use a calculator to convert each fraction to a decimal, by dividing the numerator by the denominator. $6 \div 13 = 0.4615 \ldots$, $7 \div 12 = 0.5833 \ldots$, $11 \div 16 = 0.6875$, and $9 \div 12 = 0.75$. We want to compare those with $2 \div 3 = 0.6666 \ldots$. It is evident that 0.6875 and 0.75 are greater than 0.6666..., and of the remaining two numbers, the larger is 0.5833..., or $\frac{7}{12}$.

It is possible to solve this problem without a calculator and without converting the fractions to decimals, but it is more involved. There are some shortcuts we can use if we're familiar with fractions to make some estimates that will help us, but without those shortcuts we'll have to compare each fraction to $\frac{2}{3}$, finding which ones are less than $\frac{2}{3}$ and what the difference is. To find the difference between $\frac{2}{3}$ and $\frac{6}{13}$, we can rewrite both fractions with the same denominator, $\frac{2 \times 13}{3 \times 13} = \frac{26}{39}$ and $\frac{6 \times 3}{13 \times 3} = \frac{18}{39}$. $26 > 18$, so $\frac{6}{13} < \frac{2}{3}$... so far so good. The difference is $\frac{26-18}{39} = \frac{8}{39}$. Proceeding similarly with the other numbers, we find that the difference between $\frac{2}{3}$ and $\frac{7}{12}$ is $\frac{1}{12}$, and that both $\frac{11}{16}$ and $\frac{9}{12}$ are greater than $\frac{2}{3}$, ruling these last two out as answers. So the answer must be A or B; it only remains to find which is closer to $\frac{2}{3}$—i.e. which difference is smaller. Converting them, again, to the same denominator, we get $\frac{8}{39} = \frac{8 \times 4}{39 \times 4} = \frac{32}{156}$, and $\frac{1}{12} = \frac{1 \times 13}{12 \times 13} = \frac{13}{156}$. Clearly $13 < 32$, so $\frac{1}{12} < \frac{8}{39}$, and so it is $\frac{7}{12}$ which is closer to $\frac{2}{3}$.

157. B: If $\frac{1}{3}$ of the patients seen are pediatric patients, then $\frac{1}{3}$ of the circle should indicate pediatric. The full circle contains 360 degrees, so $\frac{1}{3}$ of the circle is $\frac{1}{3}$ of 360 = 120 degrees.

158. C: The average of a series of values is equal to the total sum of the values divided by the number of values. In this case, then, to find the average weekly food expenditure we divide the total food expenditure times the number of weeks. From the given information, the total food expenditure is $\$25 + \$52 + \$52 + \$34 = \$163$. This was over four weeks, so the average weekly food expenditure was $\$163 \div 4 = \$40.75$.

159. A: We can easily solve this problem by typing the operation into a calculator. However, it's not difficult to do without a calculator, either. We just write the numbers one over the other, lining them up at the decimal point and padding the top number with zeroes on the right until it goes out to the same number of places as the bottom number:

$$\begin{array}{r} 437.650 \\ -\ 325.752 \end{array}$$

Now, we subtract the two exactly as we would subtract ordinary integers, putting the decimal point in our answer in the same place as it is in the numbers above:

$$\begin{array}{r} 6\,{}^{1}5\,{}^{1}4\,{}^{1} \\ 437.650 \\ -\ 325.752 \\ \hline 111.898 \end{array}$$

160. A: Again, we can solve this problem simply by just typing the expression into a calculator. However, it can also be done without a calculator. We can multiply these numbers just as if they were integers, ignoring the decimal points at first:

$$\begin{array}{r} 43.3 \\ \times 23.03 \\ \hline 1299 \\ 0 \\ 1299 \\ 866 \\ \hline 997199 \end{array}$$

Now, we count the total number of digits after the decimal points in the factors, and place the decimal point in the product so that it has that same number of digits after it. In this case, 43.3 has one digit after the decimal point, and 23.03 has two, so our product should have three digits after the decimal point. The answer is 997.199.

161. D: To find out how much the patient lost, we need to calculate 6% of 157. A percentage is a number of hundredths, so we can express 6% as either a fraction, $\frac{6}{100}$, or a decimal, 0.06. Either way, to find 6% of 157, we can multiply this fraction or decimal by 157: $0.06 \times 157 = 9.42$, or, rounded to the nearest pound, 9. That's the amount of weight *lost*, so to find the final weight we subtract that from the initial weight, 157: $157 - 9 = 148$.

Alternatively, we could have done the subtraction first: if the patient lost 6% of their original body weight, then their final weight was $100\% - 6\% = 94\%$ of their body weight. We then can multiply that by 157: $94\% \times 157 = 0.94 \times 157 = 147.58$, which rounds to 148.

162. B: 65% of the school's 650 students must request the vending machine. To determine how many students that is, we just multiply 65% by 650. 65% means 65 hundredths, so we can express the percentage as a fraction, $\frac{65}{100}$, or as a decimal, 0.65, and then carry out the multiplication: $0.65 \times 650 = 422.5$, which we can round up to 423.

So, we know that 423 students must request the vending machine. We are told that 340 students have already requested it. To find out how many *more* students must request the vending machine, then, we just subtract the number of students who have already requested it from the total number of students required: $423 - 340 = 83$.

163. C: The digit just before the decimal point is in the unit (ones) space, and each space right from there represents $\frac{1}{10}$ the amount of the previous space. The digit just after the decimal place is the tenths place, and the digit after that—the second digit after the decimal place—is the hundredths. This, then, is the digit we want to round to: the second digit after the decimal place, which in this case is 4. Because the next digit after that, 6, is greater than 5, we round up, so the 4 becomes a 5 and we remove all the following digits. So we're left with 390.25.

164. A: One way to solve this problem is as follows: We're asked, effectively, to solve the equation $\frac{4}{5}x = 1$. We can get the x by itself by dividing both sides by $\frac{4}{5}$: so $x = 1 \div \frac{4}{5}$. Dividing by a fraction is equivalent to multiplying by its reciprocal—the same fraction with the numerator and denominator swapped—so this is equivalent to $1 \times \frac{5}{4}$, which of course is just $\frac{5}{4}$.

However, we don't have to go to that much trouble, if we just recall that a fraction times its reciprocal is always 1. So if we want to know what number times $\frac{4}{5}$ will equal 1, the answer must be just the reciprocal of $\frac{4}{5}$, which is $\frac{5}{4}$.

165. C: The average of a series of values is equal to the total sum of the values divided by the number of values. In this case, the sum is $300 \text{ mg} + 1240 \text{ mg} + 900 \text{ mg} + 1500 \text{ mg} + 900 \text{ mg} = 4840 \text{ mg}$. This is the total over five days, so to find the average we divide this total by five: $4840 \text{ mg} \div 5 = 968 \text{ mg}$.

166. C: The tenth is the first digit after the decimal point. This rules out A, which leaves *two* digits after the decimal point, which means it's rounded to the nearest hundredth. When rounding, we round *down*—leaving the last digit as it is—if the next digit is less than 5, and we round *up*—increasing the last digit by 1—if it is 5 or greater. In choice B, the digit after the tenths digit is a 6, so the number should be rounded up: the tenths digit should be increased. But it isn't—the 5 remains a 5 rather than being changed to a 6. Conversely, in choice D, the digit after the tenths digit is a 2, so the number should be rounded down: the tenths digit should stay the same. But instead, it's incorrectly increased to 4. Choices B and D are therefore incorrect.

In choice C, the digit after the tenths digit is 8. This means we round up, the 9 changes to a 10. The 1 carries over to the next digit to the left, increasing it as well. This is exactly what we see in the answer: the 9 changes to a 0 and the 6 increases to a 7. Choice C is therefore the correct answer. As for the other answers, the number in choice A should be rounded to 3.8; choice B should be rounded to 4.6; and choice D should be rounded to 54.3.

167. C: There are several ways to approach this problem. One is to express the decimal as a fraction. Since there are three digits after the decimal point, the decimal represents a number of thousandths; the equivalent fraction is $\frac{625}{1000}$. Since both 625 and 1000 are divisible by 5, this fraction can be reduced to $\frac{625\div5}{1000\div5} = \frac{125}{200}$. Since 125 and 200 are also both divisible by 5, we can further reduce the fraction to $\frac{125\div5}{200\div5} = \frac{25}{40}$. We can still repeat the process one more time: $\frac{25\div5}{40\div5} = \frac{5}{8}$.

While this is the most straightforward way to solve the problem, we could also have done it the other way around, converting each fraction to a decimal and seeing which one matched. We can convert a fraction to a decimal by just dividing the numerator by the denominator (a calculator makes this easier, but isn't required). $\frac{3}{4} = 3 \div 4 = 0.75$, $\frac{5}{6} = 5 \div 6 = 0.8333...$, $\frac{5}{8} = 0.625$ (as desired), and $\frac{2}{3} = 0.6666...$

168. A: We can call the volume of the solution that can be made *x*. We know 6% of the solution is pure bleach. We can therefore express the amount of bleach as $6\% \times x$—or, converting the 6% into a decimal, $0.06x$. (A percentage is a number of hundredths, so we can convert a percentage to a decimal by dividing by 100—or, equivalently, by moving the decimal point two spaces to the left.) Now, the amount of pure bleach that we have is 50 mL. That means $0.06x = 50 \text{ mL}$. To solve for *x*, we can divide both sides by 0.06: $\frac{0.06x}{0.06} = \frac{50 \text{ mL}}{0.06}$, so $x = 50 \text{ mL} \div 0.06 = 833.333... \text{ mL}$, which rounds to 833 mL.

We could also have expressed the percentage as a fraction instead of a decimal: $6\% = \frac{6}{100}$, so $\frac{6}{100}x = 50 \text{ mL}$, and $x = 50 \text{ mL} \div \frac{6}{100} = 50 \text{ mL} \times \frac{100}{6} = \frac{5000 \text{ mL}}{6} = 833.333... \text{ mL}$, again rounding to 833 mL.

169. A: While we could solve this problem easily using a calculator, it's also not that hard to solve by hand. To multiply two decimal numbers, follow the same procedure as if you were multiplying two ordinary integers, ignoring the decimal point until the last step:

$$\begin{array}{r} 8.7 \\ \times\, 23.3 \\ \hline 26\ 1 \\ 261 \\ 174 \\ \hline 2027\ 1 \end{array}$$

Then, count the total number of digits after the decimal points in the two factors. The product should have that same number of digits after the decimal point. 8.7 has one digit after the decimal point, and 23.3 has one, so between them they have a total of two digits after the decimal points. So the product should also have two digits after the decimal point, and the correct answer is 202.71.

170. A: This is another problem that we could solve with a calculator, but that we could also do without a calculator if necessary. To divide a decimal number, we can perform a long division the same way as we would if we were dividing integers, placing the decimal point in the quotient directly above the decimal point in the dividend.

$$\begin{array}{r} 26.9 \\ 5\overline{)134.5} \\ 10 \\ \hline 34 \\ 30 \\ \hline 4\ 5 \\ 4\ 5 \\ \hline 0 \end{array}$$

If there had also been a decimal point in the divisor, we would have to eliminate it by moving the decimal point to the right the same number of spaces in the dividend as the number of digits after the decimal point in the divisor. In this case, however, the divisor was an integer, so that wasn't necessary.

171. C: A fraction is essentially a way to express a quotient: it's equal to the numerator divided by the denominator. So $23 \div 3$ can be written as $\frac{23}{3}$. However, this is an improper fraction—a fraction with a numerator larger than the denominator—while all the answer choices are mixed numbers—numbers consisting of an integer and a (proper) fraction.

We therefore have to convert this improper fraction into a mixed number. We do that by dividing the numerator by the denominator, making note of both the quotient and the remainder. $23 \div 3 = 7$, with a remainder of 2. The quotient is the integer in the mixed number, and the remainder is the numerator of the fraction part. So the correct answer is $7\frac{2}{3}$.

172. C: Once again, we could add these numbers with a calculator, but we could also do it by hand. We place the numbers in a column and add one place value at a time, carrying the tens digit of the sum as necessary. For example, $0 + 2 + 9 = 11$, so the rightmost digit of the answer is 1 and we carry a 1 to the next column, giving us $1 + 0 + 2 + 0 = 3$, and so on:

$$\begin{array}{r} ^{1}4^{1}500 \\ 3422 \\ +3909 \\ \hline 11831 \end{array}$$

173. C: This is a simple addition problem involving the process of carrying. Start with the ones column and add 4+7. Write down the 1 and add the 1 to the digits in the tens column: Now add 3+7+1. Write down the 1 and add the 1 to the digits in the hundreds column. Add 6+3+1 and write down 0. Add the 1 to the digits in the thousands column. Add 4+7+1 and write down the 1. Add the 1 to the digits in the ten-thousands column. Add 1+1 and write down 2 to get the answer 22,011.

174. D: This is a simple subtraction problem. Start with the ones column and subtract 5-2, then 4-3, then 6-1, then 9-6 to get 3,513.

175. D: This is a multiplication problem with carrying. Start with the ones column. Multiply 4 by each digit in above it beginning with the ones column. Write down each product: going across it will read 3572. Now multiply 6 by each of the digits above it. Write down each product: going across it will read 5358. Ensure that the 8 is in the tens column and the other numbers fall evenly to the right. Now add the numbers like a regular addition problem to get 57,152

176. A: This is a simple division problem. Divide 97 into 292. It goes in 3 times. Write 3 above the second 2 and subtract 291 from 292. The result is 1. Bring down the 9. Since 19 cannot be divided into 97, write a zero next to the 3. Bring down the 4. Drive 97 into 194. It goes 2 times.

177. A: To change this fraction into a decimal, divide 100 into 38. 100 goes into 38 0.38 times.

178. C: This is a simple addition problem. Line up the decimals so that they are all in the same place in the equation, and see that there is a 6 by itself in the hundredths column. Then add the tenths column: 8+3to get 11. Write down the 1 and carry the 1. Add the ones column: 6+1 plus the carried 1. Write down 8. Then write down the 1.

179. D: This is multiplication with decimals. Multiply the 7 by 8 to get 56. Put down the 6 and carry the 5. Multiply 7 by 2 to get 14. Add the 5. Write 19 to left of 6. Multiply the 1 by the 8 to get 8. Multiply 1 by 2 to get 2. Add the two lines together, making sure that the 8 in the bottom figure is even with the 9. Get 476. Count 4 decimal points over (2 from the top multiplier and 2 from the second multiplier) and add a 0 before adding the decimal.

180. C: Count from the 3: tenths, hundredths, thousandths.

181. A: Write 512 then add the decimal in the thousandths place, the third place from the right.

182. A: To add fractions, ensure that the denominator (the number on the bottom) is the same. Since it is not, change them both to 56ths. $\frac{1}{8} = \frac{7}{56}; \frac{3}{7} = \frac{24}{56}$. Now add the whole numbers: $3 + 6 = 9$ and the fractions $\frac{7}{56} + \frac{24}{56} = \frac{31}{56}$.

183. C: To subtract fractions, ensure that the denominator (the number on the bottom) is the same. Since it is not, change them both to 14ths. $\frac{1}{7} = \frac{2}{14}; \frac{1}{2} = \frac{7}{14}$. The equation now looks like this: $4\frac{2}{14} -$

$2\frac{7}{14}$. Change the 4 to 3 and add 14 to the numerator (the top number) so that the fractions can be subtracted. The equation now looks like this: $3\frac{16}{14} - 2\frac{7}{14}$. Subtract: $1\frac{9}{14}$

184. A: To multiply mixed numbers, first create improper fractions. Multiply the whole number by the denominator, then add the numerator. $1\frac{1}{4}$ becomes $\frac{5}{4}$; $3\frac{2}{5}$ becomes $\frac{17}{5}$; $1\frac{2}{3}$ becomes $\frac{5}{3}$.

The problem will look like this: $\frac{5}{4} \times \frac{17}{5} \times \frac{5}{3} = \frac{425}{60} = 7\frac{5}{60} = 7\frac{1}{12}$.

185. A: To divide fractions, change the second fraction to its reciprocal (its reverse) and multiply: $\frac{3}{5} \times \frac{2}{1}$

186. A: To solve, test each answer. Notice that in (A), the numerator has been multiplied by 3 to get 12. The denominator has been multiplied by 3 to get 21. In (B) the numerator has been multiplied by 4 and the denominator has been multiplied by 5. In (C), the numerator has been multiplied by 3 and the denominator has been multiplied by 4. In (D), the numerator has been multiplied by 4 and the denominator has been multiplied by a number less than 4.

187. D: To solve for *n*, begin by cross-multiplying:

$$21 \times n = 7 \times 18$$

$$21n = 126$$

$$n = 6$$

Alternatively, notice that 7 is $21 \div 3$ and divide 18 by 3 to find *n*.

188. C: If 98 is divisible by 14, dividing both numerator and denominator by 14 will automatically provide you with the lowest possible terms.

$$\frac{14 \div 14}{98 \div 14} = \frac{1}{7}$$

189. A: To convert an improper fraction to a mixed number, divide the numerator by the denominator and note the whole number and remainder that result:

$$68 \div 7 = 9.7143 \ldots$$

$$9 \times 7 = 63$$

$$68 - 63 = 5$$

So 68 divided by 7 is 9 with a remainder of 5. Thus, the equivalent mixed number is $9\frac{5}{7}$.

190. A: Since a percentage is by definition a number of hundredths, thirty-six hundredths is necessarily the same as 36%.

191. A: Set up the equation as follows:

$$x \times 60 = 3$$

$$x = \frac{3}{60} = \frac{1}{20} = 5\%$$

192. D: Set up the equation as follows:

$$x \times 25 = 1$$

$$x = \frac{1}{25} = 4\%$$

193. A: Set up the equation as follows:

$$x = \frac{3}{8} \times 40$$

$$x = \frac{120}{8} = 15$$

194. D: To solve, first get both fractions on the same side of the equation to isolate the percentage sign. When $\frac{5}{6}$ is moved to the opposite side of the equation, it must be divided by the fraction there: $\frac{1}{3} \div \frac{5}{6}$ To divide one fraction into another, multiply by the reciprocal of the denominator:

$$\frac{1}{3} \times \frac{6}{5} = \frac{6}{15} = \frac{2}{5} = 40\%$$

195. D: Since we know that 3 represents the part and 15 represents the whole, we can consider the ratio as a simple fraction: $\frac{3}{15}$. This can be reduced by dividing numerator and denominator by 3, leaving us with $\frac{1}{5}$, which is equivalent to 20%.

196. C: To convert a fraction to a percentage, first check whether the denominator is a factor of 100 (2, 4, 5, 10, 20, 25, or 50). If it is not, reduce the fraction as far as possible and check again. Then manipulate so that the denominator is 100:

$$\frac{3 \div 3}{12 \div 3} = \frac{1}{4}$$

$$\frac{1 \times 25}{4 \times 25} = \frac{25}{100} = 25\%$$

197. D: Since a percentage is equivalent to a fraction with a denominator of 100, 8% can be rewritten as $\frac{8}{100}$. Reduce the fraction as far as possible by dividing by common factors:

$$\frac{8 \div 4}{100 \div 4} = \frac{2}{25}$$

Biology

198. A: Sodium and potassium are the two key ingredients needed to transmit a message down the nerve cell. The ions move in and out of the cell to generate an action potential to convey the impulse. Once the impulse reaches the end of the neuron, calcium channels open to allow calcium to rush into the synaptic space. Actin and myosin are the two proteins that cause contraction of muscle fibers.

199. B: The answer is translocation. Nondisjunction is a genetic mutation where the chromosomes fail to separate after replication. This results in two cells with an abnormal number of chromosomes (one with too many, one with too few). Deletion is when a section of the chromosome is erased. Crossing over occurs when the two chromosomes are joined by the centromere and two of the legs cross over and switch places on the two chromosomes.

200. A: Our skin and mucus membranes are the first line of defense against potentially invading bacteria. Their purpose is to keep the bacteria from getting into the body in the first place. Any break or tear in the skin or mucus membranes can allow harmful bacteria or viruses to attack the body. Once inside, macrophages, T-cells, and lymphocytes will be summoned to attack infected body cells and the invading pathogens.

201. C: Capping the end of a mRNA strand protects the strand from degradation and "wear and tear." Such damage to a strand of mRNA could be catastrophic, as it directs the synthesis of proteins that are vital for life.

202. A: A clue here is that chlorophyll is involved, meaning this is a photosynthesis reaction. The light-dependent reaction involves a hydrolysis reaction to provide electrons to chlorophyll, and the release of oxygen molecules. During the light-independent reaction, the energy produced from the dependent reaction is stored in the form of chemical bonds in glucose molecules.

203. D: Photosynthesis is the process that plant cells use to obtain energy from the sun. Diffusion and active transport are both methods of ionic movement, but transpiration occurs when water moves up a plant's conduction tubes against the force of gravity.

204. C: Ethylene is the plant hormone that causes ripening of fruit. Auxins and cytokinins both promote cell growth. Auxins specifically encourage stem elongation and can also inhibit growth of lateral branches. Abscisic acid inhibits cell growth and seed germination.

205. D: Thigmotropism is the growth of plant structures in response to physical contact, similar to how vines will change their direction of growth to stay in contact with a wall or other item. Growth towards light is called phototropism, and gravitropism is growth of leaves and stems opposite to the force of gravity.

206. A: The stigma is a long tube that extends from the center of a flower whose function it is to gather pollen and transport it down the carpel toward the ovum. The bright colored petals of a flower help attract pollinators like birds, bees, and butterflies. Pollen is made in the stamen and anther, which protrude from the flower to make it easier for the pollinators to gather pollen as they fly from flower to flower. The ovary of the flower provides nourishment for the developing seeds.

207. B: Think of the mnemonic "Dear King Philip Came Over For Good Soup." This stands for domain, kingdom, phylum, class, order, family, genus, species. It relates the classification system for every species organism in the world. The further down the line that two species are similar, the more closely related they are. Genus is the most specific taxonomic category listed in the given answer choices, and so organisms with the same genus are most closely related.

208. B: A pioneer species is the first species to colonize a new area. Primary producers are organisms that produce their own food, usually from sunlight. Primary producers tend to be plants. Primary consumers are herbivores and eat primary producers. Secondary consumers eat primary consumers, and tertiary consumers eat secondary consumers.

209. C: Microtubules, microfilaments and intermediate filaments are all types of fibrous proteins that are found in the cytoskeleton and provide structural support. They also assist in the transport of materials and aid in cell motility. Glycoproteins are not found in the cytoskeleton.

210. D: Coniferous forests are populated by cone-bearing trees, or conifers. Tundra are very cold and harsh environments located mainly in the arctic. These biomes are characterized by very low temperatures and harsh winds. Tropical forests have a very dense population of different tree and plant species, with varying amounts of precipitation, and tend to exist around the equator. Temperate deciduous forests are found in moderate climates where there are warm summers and cold winters. During the winters, the trees will lose their leaves.

211. B: Biotic factors are living things, like plants and animals. Populations, communities, and individuals are also examples of biotic factors. The most basic abiotic factors are temperature, water, sunlight, and wind.

212. D: Detritivores eat only dead and decaying matter Herbivores eat plants, carnivores eat meat, and omnivores eat both plants and animals.

213. A: This type of growth produces an S curve, similar to "∫". Look at the shape and you can see how it starts out with a slow rise and then increases dramatically. After a rapid period of growth, the curve levels off at the top of the S shape.

214. C: When one member of a symbiotic relationship benefits and the other is harmed, it is termed parasitism. Mutualism occurs when both members benefit from the symbiotic relationship. Predation is when one member actively feeds on the other, causing death of the hunted species. During commensalism, one member of the relationship benefits and the other neither benefits nor is harmed.

215. A: The genotype for the two parents is Bb. Crossing Bb with Bb will give 75% brown mice and 25% white mice. Twenty-five percent of 24 is six white mice.

216. C: The genotype for each of the parents is RrWw. Set up a Punnett Square for the cross RrWw X RrWw. There are 16 possible outcomes: nine red eyes with wings: three red eyes without wings: three white eyes with wings: one white eye without wings.

217. B: Sex linked traits are carried on the X chromosome, which means that men are significantly more affected than women. Affected men can inherit the trait from either parent, depending on who carries the gene. Such disorders can occur in females—if both parents carry the trait and pass it on to their daughter—but it is very rare.

218. D: Prokaryotic cells are single-celled organisms that don't have a formal nucleus. Pili and flagella are external structures that help the cell move around. Pili are a small arm-like protrusion that can stick to other surfaces; flagella are long whip-like structures that move in a rapid fashion to propel the cell forward. A capsule is a sticky coating that some cells secrete to help the cell stick to a surface and can even provide some degree of protection. Most cells have a rigid outer cell wall (external to the plasma membrane) that provides a great deal of protection for the cell.

219. A: Enzymes are proteins that facilitate reactions, making it easier or even possible for the reaction to occur. There are several factors that can affect how well the enzyme functions: temperature, pH of the environment, and concentration of the enzyme or substrate. In addition, the presence of other proteins, called competitive or noncompetitive inhibitors will have a direct impact on enzymatic function.

220. B: The process of transcription is the conversion of DNA into mRNA, which is a complementary form of the original DNA strand. That means that mRNA is formed with the opposite bases. For example, a DNA strand of CGATGA would form an mRNA strand of GCUACU. In RNA, the base uracil is used instead of thymine. Transcription allows the ribosome to read the information coded in DNA to form proteins.

221. C: Translation is the process of reading a strand of mRNA and assembling the amino acid chain according to the information encoded on that strand. This process takes place in the ribosome.

222. D: Stabilizing selection occurs when the intermediate form of a trait, rather than the extreme form, is being selected for. Directional evolution tends to favor one of the extreme forms of the trait so that eventually, the trait typically becomes more apparent and more extreme as time goes on. Both convergent and divergent evolution refers to patterns of evolution among groups of species. Divergent evolution occurs when groups of species with a common ancestral trait evolve into different adaptations over time. Convergent evolution refers to when species that aren't related to each other develop similar traits independently of each other.

Chemistry

223. C: Use the equation, $[H^+] = 10^{-pH}$, to find that the concentration of hydrogen ions is 10^{-7}. The pH of a neutral solution is 7.

224. B: Adding an acid to a base will always yield water and a salt. It is difficult to determine the pH of the resulting solution because it depends on how acidic and basic the two initial solutions are.

225. D: Alcohols are classified by the presence of a hydroxyl group (oxygen bound to a hydrogen atom). Compounds with nitrogen bonded to other carbon atoms are called amines and are further classified according to how many carbons are attached to the nitrogen. A carbon atom with a double bond to an oxygen atom and a single bond to a hydroxyl group is the functional group of carboxylic acids. Benzene rings are an example of an aromatic hydrocarbon.

226. B: Amines are classified by the number of carbon atoms the nitrogen is bonded to. In a primary amine, nitrogen is bound to one carbon (designated by R functional group). In secondary and tertiary amines, the nitrogen is bound to two and three carbons respectively. Choice A is an example of a ketone.

227. D: Hydrocarbons are a class of molecules that contain only hydrogen and carbon. They tend to be volatile and reactive, with low boiling and melting points. London dispersion forces are present in every molecule, and hydrocarbons are no exception. Hydrocarbons tend to be gases at room temperature, not solids.

228. A: Ketones and aldehydes are very similar structurally. They each have a double bond between carbon and oxygen. In ketones, there are two functional bonds to the central carbon, while in aldehydes there is only one functional group and a hydrogen atom bound to the central carbon. They both have some properties of nonpolar and polar compounds.

229. C: A substitution reaction occurs in hydrocarbons when one of the hydrogen atoms is replaced with a different atom. When a radical, or highly reactive compound or atom, reacts with and bonds to an unpaired electron in any open shell, it is called a radical reaction. Hydrolysis and condensation are almost exactly opposite. Hydrolysis refers to when a water molecule is added to a compound to break it apart. Condensation occurs when water is released after two groups bond together.

230. D: These are called resonance structures. The double bond can occupy any of these positions and rather than alternate between these three different structures, the molecule is actually a hybrid of all three at once. It is said that there are three 1 ⅓ bonds between the oxygen and nitrogen molecules.

231. B: Positron emission and electron capture are both examples of radioactive decay processes, which release radioactive particles. Using these theories of radioactive decay can lead to extreme energy production. Nuclear fission is the process when a neutron bombards and splits open a nucleus. Fusion occurs when hydrogen atoms combine to form helium and electrons, releasing a tremendous amount of energy, far more than fission reactions.

232. D: The noble gases, group 18 on the periodic table, have a full valence shell of 8 electrons. This is significant because it means that the gases are completely inert and unable to form compounds with other elements.

233. A: This is Avogadro's number, and needs to be memorized. One mole is 6.022×10^{23} units of anything. It is a commonly used constant.

234. B: To convert from Fahrenheit to Celsius, simply subtract 32 from the Fahrenheit temperature and divide the result by 1.8. Next, to convert from Celsius to Kelvin, add 273 to the Celsius temperature. 99.1^{o} F = 37° C = 310 Kelvin.

235. B: Start this problem by converting the temperatures to Kelvin: $35°\text{C} = (273.15 + 35)$ K and $100°\text{C} = (273.15 + 100)$ K. Use Gay-Lussac's law: $\frac{P_1}{T_1} = \frac{P_2}{T_2}$. Solving for the initial pressure: $P_1 = \frac{P_2T_1}{T_2} = \frac{(2.5\text{ atm})(308.15\text{ K})}{373.15\text{ K}} = 2.1$ atm.

236. C: According to the ideal gas law, PV = nRT, the pressure of the gas will decrease as the volume increases. This is because there will be the same amount of gas but in a larger space. According to Charles' Law, temperature and volume are directly related. This means that as the volume of the gas increases, the temperature of the gas will increase as well. Increasing the volume of the gas will have no effect on the number of moles or volatility.

237. D: A covalent bond forms between two atoms when the electron pair forming the bond are shared between the two atoms. When both shared electrons come from the same atom, it is called a coordinate covalent bond. An ionic bond forms when one electron is actually transferred from one atom to the other during the process.

238. B: During a combustion reaction, light and heat are released as water and carbon dioxide are formed. It is a rapid and often violent reaction that usually occurs in the presence of oxygen.

239. C: Colligative properties are properties that depend on the amount of solute in a solution. The elevation of a solution's boiling point, depression of its freezing point, and vapor pressure are all examples of a colligative property. If solute is added to the solution, the degree of depression or elevation changes in relation to the amount of solute added.

240. D: To balance the carbon atoms in the above equation, you must place a 6 in front of the molecule of CO_2. A 6 must also be placed in front of the molecule of water to balance the hydrogen atoms. Finally, there are 18 atoms of oxygen on the right side of the equation. On the left, there are 6 atoms in the glucose molecule, so by placing a 6 in front of the oxygen molecule, the equation will be balanced.

241. B: There are three laws of thermodynamics. The first is that energy is finite and is neither created nor destroyed. The second law is that entropy, or disorder, is always increasing in the universe. The third, and final, law of thermodynamics is that there is no disorder or entropy when a perfect crystal is at absolute zero temperature. Choice D is not one of the laws of thermodynamics.

242. D: When two atoms are bonded together, they share an electron pair, or two electrons. If a double bond is formed, they share two pairs of electrons, or four electrons. Three electrons pairs or six electrons are shared in a triple bond.

243. A: When it comes to their reaction to water, molecules are either hydrophobic or hydrophilic. Hydrophobic molecules are 'afraid' (think: phobic) of water, and tend to be nonpolar and cluster together to minimize their contact with water. Hydrophilic, or water-loving, molecules are usually polar because of their ability to react with other charged molecules.

244. C: A monosaccharide is a single sugar molecule, with the basic formula of $(CH_2O)_N$ Glucose, fructose, and mannose are all examples of monosaccharides. Sucrose is a disaccharide—two sugar molecules linked together.

245. B: An exergonic reaction is one that releases energy or heat, such as combustion. These reactions tend to occur spontaneously. An endergonic reaction is one that absorbs energy and thus cannot occur unless energy is available to feed the reaction A hydrolysis reaction refers to one where a molecule of water is added across a molecule to break the molecular bonds.

246. C: There are several different ways to classify acids and bases. According to the Arrhenius definition, acids give off hydrogen ions (H^+) in a solution and bases give off hydroxide ions (OH^-) in a solution. According to the Brønsted-Lowery definition, acids also donate protons (H^+) but bases accept the protons. The Lewis definition is another classification of acids/bases, where acids have the ability to accept a pair of electrons, while the base is able to donate a pair of electrons.

247. A: London dispersion forces are weak forces that exist between all molecules and, in fact, are the only forces that are present in some compounds, such as nonpolar molecules. Dipole-dipole forces are present in dipolar compounds, which govern the behavior of these substances. There are no such forces as hydrogen forces, though hydrogen bonding occurs between hydrogen atoms and either nitrogen, oxygen, or fluorine, which form very polar compounds. Chemical bonds are the forces that bond atoms to each other and are not an example of an intermolecular force.

Anatomy and Physiology

248. B: The reticular activating system (RAS) is primarily responsible for the arousal and maintenance of consciousness. The midbrain is a part of the brainstem, which has a crucial role in the regulation of autonomic functions like breathing and heart rate. The diencephalon consists of the hypothalamus and thalamus in the middle part of the brain between the cerebrum and midbrain. It plays a huge role in regulating and coordinating sensory information and hormonal secretion from the hypothalamus. The limbic system tends to the major instinctual drives like eating, sex, thirst, and aggression.

249. A: The triceps reflex forces the triceps to contract, which in turn extends the arm. Eliciting the deep tendon reflexes is an important indication of neural functioning. Without them, it can be a clue to serious spinal cord or other neurological injury. The physician should be notified immediately if a patient loses deep tendon reflexes.

250. C: The acoustic nerve, or CN VIII, is responsible for hearing and balance. To test this nerve, the practitioner could test the patient's hearing in each ear and use a tuning fork to determine the patient's ability to hear and feel the vibrations.

251. A: The parathyroid glands are four small glands that sit on top of the thyroid gland and regulate calcium levels by secreting parathyroid hormone. The hormone regulates the amount of calcium and magnesium that is excreted by the kidneys into the urine.

252. D: The empty egg follicle (once the egg was ovulated) is now called the corpus luteum and secretes large amounts of progesterone. Progesterone is the primary hormone responsible for maintaining a pregnancy. Follicle stimulating hormone and luteinizing hormone have already stopped production, and estrogen decreased right before ovulation.

253. B: Insulin and glucagon are the two main options here. Insulin is produced during periods of high blood sugar and promotes glucose absorption into the cells and the storage of glucose as glycogen and lipids in the liver. Glucagon has the opposite effect; when blood sugar is low, glucagon production promotes the breakdown of glycogen into glucose.

254. D: The myocardium is the layer of the heart that contains the muscle fibers responsible for contraction (Hint: myo- is the prefix for muscle). The endocardium and epicardium are the inner and outer layers of the heart wall, respectively. The pericardium is the sac in which the heart sits inside the chest cavity.

255. C: The SA node in the right atrium generates the impulse that travels through the heart tissue and to the AV node. The AV node sits in the wall of the right atrium and coordinates atrial and ventricular contraction of the heart. The impulse then travels down to the bundle of His, the two main (left and right) branches of conduction fibers and to the Purkinje fibers which spread the impulse throughout the rest of the heart.

256. A: This is a tricky question; most of the time, veins carry deoxygenated blood and arteries carry oxygenated blood. However, in this case, the pulmonary veins carry oxygenated blood from the lungs to the heart and the pulmonary arteries carry deoxygenated blood from the heart to the lungs.

257. C: Eosinophils are most commonly recruited to deal with allergenic antigens. Monocytes, neutrophils, and basophils also deal with antigens during the immune response, but eosinophils are found to be elevated during an allergic response.

258. B: Vitamin K is stored by the liver and is essential for the synthesis and conversion of several clotting factors, including Factor II, Factor VII, Factor IX, and Factor X. Without adequate amounts of this vitamin, the clotting factors will not be able to function properly.

259. C: Afferent vessels carry fluid toward a structure; efferent vessels carry fluid away from the structure. So afferent lymph vessels carry lymph towards the node, and efferent vessels carry lymph away from the node.

260. D: Cricoid cartilage refers to the thick rings of cartilage that surround the trachea, sitting right above the voice box. The purpose of these thick rings is to serve as additional support and protection for the delicate airway.

261. A: The mediastinum is found in the middle of the thorax, right between the lungs. It contains many structures, including the heart, the upper part of the aorta, pulmonary blood vessels, the superior and inferior vena cava, the thymus, the trachea, the esophagus, and large nerves, such as the phrenic, vagus, and cardiac. The xiphoid process lies below the mediastinum.

262. C: The duodenum is the first segment of the small intestine, connecting to the stomach on one end and to the jejunum on the other. The jejunum sits between the duodenum and the last section of small intestine, the ileum, which then connects to the large intestine.

263. D: There are several hormones secreted in the GI system that play a role in digestion. Gastrin encourages the secretion of other gastric enzymes and the motility of the stomach, while gastric inhibitory peptides work to inhibit gastric enzymes and motility. Secretin and cholecystokinin both stimulate the release of pancreatic enzymes and peptides that are instrumental in digestion.

264. C: Food enters the digestive system through the mouth and proceeds down to the stomach after mastication by the teeth. Once in the stomach, enzymes are secreted that begin to digest the specific substances in the food (proteins, carbohydrates, etc). Next, the food passes through to the small intestine where the nutrients are absorbed and then into the large intestine where extra water is absorbed.

265. A: The bladder capacity of an average adult is approximately 500 to 600 ml. Excess urine in the bladder would eventually cause bladder distention and the back-up of urine into the rest of the urinary system.

266. C: Anti-diuretic hormone regulates the amount of urine output from the body. When ADH is produced in large amounts, the kidneys absorb extra water, concentrating the urine. When ADH secretion slows down, the kidneys release extra water and dilute the urine.

267. B: Interstitial fluid is found in the tissues around the cells; intracellular fluid is found within the cells. Fluid in the ventricles of the brain and down into the spinal cord is called cerebrospinal fluid. Cerebrospinal fluid bathes these sensitive tissues in a fluid that helps to protect them. Blood and lymph are the fluids that carry nutrients, oxygen, waste, and lymph material throughout the body.

268. D: There is a very narrow range of normal pH values in the human body, 7.35 to 7.45. Values lower than 7.35 indicate acidosis, and pHs higher than 7.45 indicate alkalosis. The human body can't function properly if the pH is outside of the normal range.

269. A: Patients with low respiratory rate or who are retaining CO_2 are at a high risk for developing respiratory acidosis. The buildup of CO_2 will lead to an elevated $PaCO_2$. Extra CO_2 in the blood will combine with water to form carbonic acid H_2CO_3, which will disassociate to form H^+ and HCO_3-. The excess hydrogen will drop the pH. If the H_2CO_3 is also abnormal and the pH is on the low side of normal, the metabolic system is likely compensating for the respiratory abnormality. This is called "compensated respiratory acidosis."

270. B: Leydig's cells, found in the testes, secrete testosterone, which is responsible for the majority of male sexual development. Sertoli cells are also in the testes but aid in supporting developing sperm cells. Skene's glands are found in the female and are not involved in testosterone production. Cowper's glands are accessory organs that secrete fluid contributing to the seminal fluid.

271. D: Every month during a normal menstrual cycle, a single egg is released from the ovary and moves down the fallopian tubes toward the uterus. If sperm cells are in the reproductive tract, they will encounter and fertilize the egg in the fallopian tubes. The fertilized egg will subsequently travel the rest of the way into the uterus and implant in the uterine lining.

272. D: Langerhans cells and melanocytes both have protective functions, though melanocytes protect the skin against UVA and UVB radiation. Langerhans cells are found in the epidermis and assist lymphocytes in processing foreign antigens. Eccrine glands secrete sweat, which aids in temperature regulation and excretion of water and electrolytes. Reticular fibers make up part of the structure of the extracellular material.

Thank You

We at Mometrix would like to extend our heartfelt thanks to you, our friend and patron, for allowing us to play a part in your journey. It is a privilege to serve people from all walks of life who are unified in their commitment to building the best future they can for themselves.

The preparation you devote to these important testing milestones may be the most valuable educational opportunity you have for making a real difference in your life. We encourage you to put your heart into it—that feeling of succeeding, overcoming, and yes, conquering will be well worth the hours you've invested.

We want to hear your story, your struggles and your successes, and if you see any opportunities for us to improve our materials so we can help others even more effectively in the future, please share that with us as well. **The team at Mometrix would be absolutely thrilled to hear from you!** So please, send us an email (support@mometrix.com) and let's stay in touch.

If you feel as though you need additional help, please check out the other resources we offer:

Study Guide: http://MometrixStudyGuides.com/HESI

Flashcards: http://MometrixFlashcards.com/HESI

Made in the USA
Monee, IL
09 December 2020

51412554R00094